# How To Conquer

# Arthritis

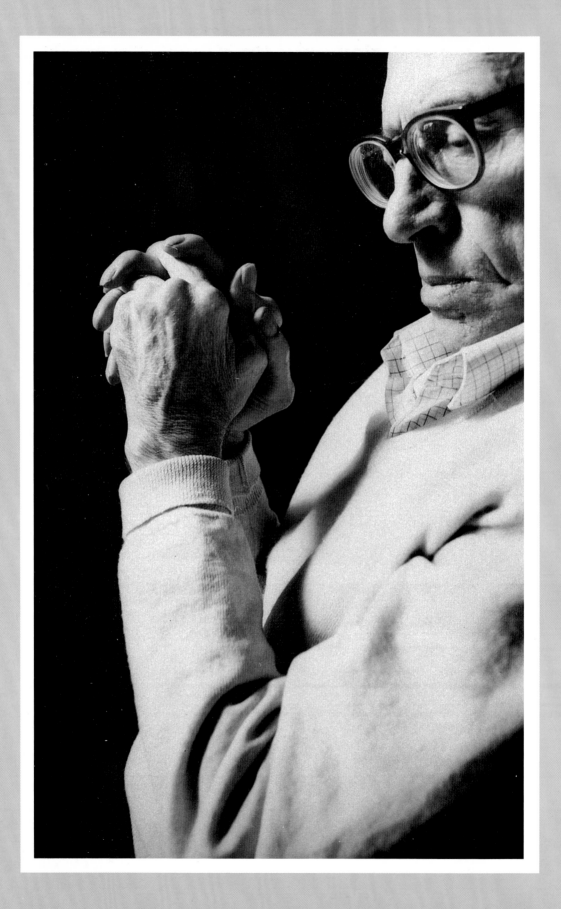

a consultation with **DR VERNON COLEMAN**

# HOW TO CONQUER ARTHRITIS

HAMLYN

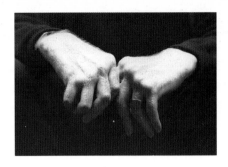

First published in Great Britain 1993
by Hamlyn, an imprint of Reed Consumer Books Limited,
Michelin House, 81 Fulham Road, London SW3 6RB
and Auckland, Melbourne, Singapore and Toronto

Copyright © Vernon Coleman 1993
Design and Illustrations © Reed International Books Limited 1993

ISBN 0 600 57577 2

A CIP record for this book is available at the British Library

Printed in Italy

# CONTENTS

# CHAPTER ONE

# What is Arthritis?

*The word 'arthritis' is often used as though it referred to a single disease – but it is about as specific as the word 'infection'. If your doctor tells you that you have arthritis he is simply telling you that you have a disease in which your joints are involved.*

## TYPES OF ARTHRITIS

Just as there are over 100 different types of infection, so there are over 100 different types of arthritis. They differ enormously in the speed with which they develop, the length of time they last and the amount and extent of damage and crippling that they do. Rheumatoid arthritis and osteoarthritis are both types of arthritis but they are as different from one another as are malaria and tuberculosis – both of which are types of infection. Arthritis is so common that most of us will suffer from at least one sort of it at least once in our lives. And, because most varieties of arthritis are incurable, once the disease has developed it often lasts for life.

Few diseases affect as many people as the diseases in the arthritis group; few cause as much pain, discomfort and disablement and few are the subject of so many myths and so much misunderstanding as to their nature.

The longer you live the more likely you are to suffer from arthritis. No matter whether you have an active life or a quiet life, there will be a type of arthritis that will, sooner or later, affect you to some degree or another.

That is, as they say, the bad news.

The good news is that although arthritic diseases are normally incurable the symptoms can usually be controlled. Arthritic diseases do not usually kill and if they are treated with care and respect the amount of damage and pain they cause can be minimized.

Just a few years ago arthritis sufferers faced a lifetime of disablement and more or less constant pain. Doctors still haven't found a 'cure' for arthritis – any more than they have found a 'cure' for infection – but they have acquired a good deal of information which should help you to stop your joints being destroyed, to relieve joint pain and stiffness, to restore lost joint function and to slow down – or even halt – the rate at which the arthritis spreads. Some arthritis treatments are, it is true, potentially hazardous, but many millions of patients around the world have been treated safely and effectively and have learned how to combat their disease.

Whether your arthritis has been caused by ageing, strain, wear and tear, an infection with a bacteria or a virus, an injury, a metabolic or a chemical abnormality, a hormonal abnormality or an immune system problem there will be things that you can do to protect yourself, to maintain your mobility and to keep your pain and stiffness to a minimum.

If the symptoms of arthritis are left untreated – or are treated half-heartedly – then they will invariably get worse. The damage that is done may eventually be irreparable. If, on the other hand, treatment is initiated early and with enthusiasm then, undoubtedly, the outlook can be greatly improved.

There are nearly 200 different joints in the human body. Your joints have a dual purpose; they make it possible for you to move, and they absorb sudden shocks (such as when you jump up in the air and land on a hard surface).

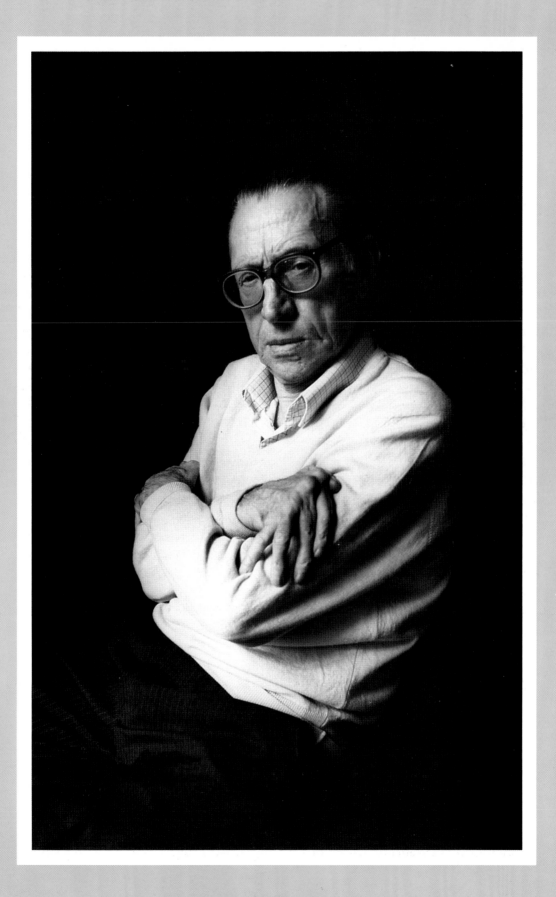

Joints can repair themselves when they are injured or damaged and they can replenish their own supplies of synovial – or lubricating – fluid.

Each joint consists of two opposing bones and on the end of each bone there is a layer of cartilage which is covered with a capsule and kept moist with a special lubricating fluid. Tendons attached to the two opposing bones help to hold the joint in position.

Joints, like every other part of your body, can become diseased, injured or infected. Indeed, there are well over 100 different joint diseases already known and the chances are that there are quite a few more still to be identified.

## THE DISEASES THAT AFFECT JOINTS FALL INTO SIX BASIC CATEGORIES

**1.** There are the inflammatory joint disorders in which the synovial membrane (which is responsible for producing the synovial fluid) becomes red and swollen. The result is that the whole joint becomes red, painful and swollen, and feels hot. If the disease is allowed to continue uncontrolled the joint will eventually be destroyed. The commonest of these disorders is rheumatoid arthritis.

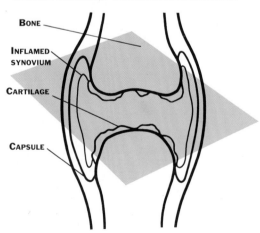

*Inflammatory joint disorder*

**2.** There are the types of disease caused by 'wear and tear' in which the cartilage covering the end of the bones wears away, leaving bone rubbing on bone. In these diseases –

known as 'degenerative' – the joints involved gradually become stiff, painful and difficult to move. The most common disorder is osteoarthritis, although the disease itself is ill-named for it is not, as its name suggests, an inflammatory disease at all. Really, osteoarthritis should be called osteoarthrosis but to avoid confusion the more common name is used here. Because it is usually caused by wear and tear, osteoarthritis is more common among the elderly.

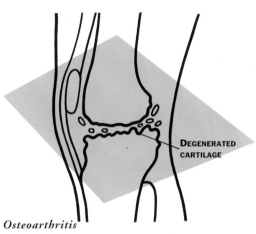

*Osteoarthritis*

**3.** There is the type of arthritis in which the inflammation occurs not in or around the synovial membrane but in the area where the ligaments and tendons join the bones. The best-known serious disease in this category is probably ankylosing spondylitis which is,

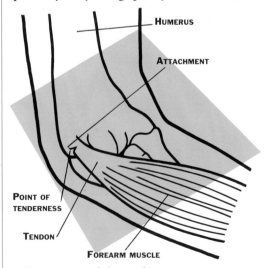

*Inflammation of the tendon*

after rheumatoid arthritis and osteoarthritis, the third commonest type of arthritis. Disorders in this general category are usually known as 'periarticular'. Tennis elbow (in which the insertion of the tendon into the bone is damaged) and housemaid's knee (in which a bursa – a small fluid-filled sac – at the knee joint is damaged and swollen) are other diseases which fall within this group.

4. There are some types of joint disease in which the problems are caused by the development of crystals within the joint. The best-known disease in this category is undoubtedly gout, in which the pain is caused by the formation of uric acid crystals in the joint space.

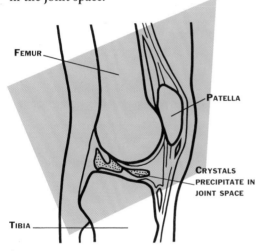

FEMUR

PATELLA

CRYSTALS PRECIPITATE IN JOINT SPACE

TIBIA

*A joint affected by uric acid crystals*

5. There are some types of arthritis known as 'infective', where organisms such as bacteria or viruses get into the joints. The symptoms of infective arthritis can develop quite quickly and the pain can be severe.

6. This type of arthritic disease does not involve the bones or joints directly but the muscles that surround a joint. It is not, therefore, a true form of arthritis. When muscles are inflamed or strained the resulting symptoms can be very similar to arthritis of the joint itself. Many types of backache fall into this category, as does fibrositis – also known as 'muscular rheumatism'.

## HOW YOUR JOINTS ARE DESIGNED

Bones are the framework upon which the rest of your body is built. They have to be very strong (bone is one of the toughest and most resilient materials known to man) and rigid. Bones are made of living tissue – they have a blood supply just like other parts of your body – and they are capable of changing their shape if your body is short of essential minerals such as calcium or if there is a constant need for extra strength in one particular area.

Joints are the junctions between bones and without them you would be unable to bend or to move around at all. Muscles which are attached to your bones produce movement by contracting (and then relaxing again) but it is your joints which make all movement possible.

If your joints simply consisted of the ends of two bones resting on one another every movement you made would be stiff, painful and

• THE BONES OF YOUR UPPER AND LOWER LEG GIVE YOUR LEGS BASIC STRENGTH BUT IT IS YOUR HIP, KNEE AND ANKLE JOINTS WHICH ENABLE YOU TO WALK, RUN, SKIP AND HOP.

• YOUR SHOULDER, ELBOW AND WRIST JOINTS ENABLE YOU TO MOVE YOUR ARMS ABOUT.

• THE SMALL JOINTS IN YOUR HAND ENABLE YOU TO PICK UP AND HOLD A PEN, A PAINTBRUSH OR A KNIFE AND FORK.

• THE JOINTS BETWEEN YOUR SKULL AND THE TOP OF YOUR SPINE ENABLE YOU TO BEND YOUR HEAD UP AND DOWN AND TO TURN IT FROM SIDE TO SIDE.

• THE INTERVERTEBRAL JOINTS WITHIN YOUR SPINE ENABLE YOU TO BEND YOUR BACK.

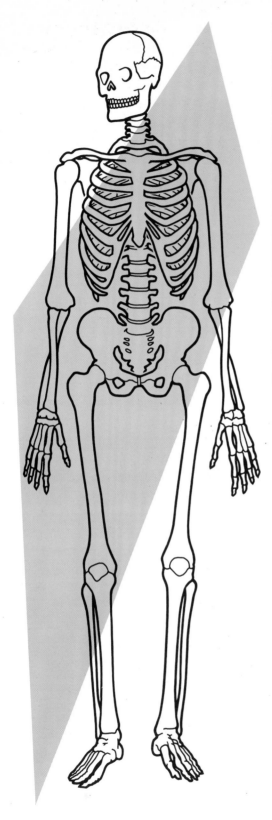

noisy. When you ran the shock of hitting the ground would be transmitted up through every bone and joint in your body. The friction between the bones of your lower leg and upper leg would be so great that every movement of your knee would be slow and difficult.

There are three types of joint in your body: synovial, fibrous and cartilaginous.

## SYNOVIAL JOINTS

In order to reduce the friction between the bones, the end of each bone is covered with a layer of cartilage – a tough, white, gristly substance which allows the bone ends to move smoothly on one another. There is less friction between two cartilaginous surfaces than there is between an ice skate and a skating rink!

Around the outside of each joint there is a membrane – called the synovium – which regularly produces a small amount of a sticky substance called synovial fluid. This fluid helps to keep the cartilage in good condition and also acts as a lubricating fluid. If the synovial membrane becomes inflamed it may start to produce too much synovial fluid or synovial fluid of the wrong consistency.

Covering the membrane or synovium is the joint capsule, which is thicker and tougher than the synovium and is designed to seal and protect the joint. In larger joints which have to carry a

*The spine is the central part of the skeleton; the skull is balanced on top of it.*

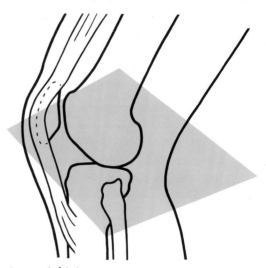

*A synovial joint*

lot of weight, the capsule contains thicker fibres called ligaments which give the joint extra stability and control the amount of movement.

The muscles that govern the movement of your body are attached to your bones by tendons. The tendons are usually attached to the end of the bones so that they can get the maximum amount of leverage. Tendons are fairly easily damaged, particularly at their thinnest point where they are attached to bone. Sudden or difficult movements can tear a tendon. When a tendon runs very close to a joint or bone, the two may rub against one another, and there will probably be a small bursa – or fluid-filled sac – to help reduce the amount of friction. If a bursa becomes inflamed it may produce too much fluid and become swollen.

## FIBROUS JOINTS

Not all joints require the full range of movement provided by a synovial membrane, synovial fluid and joint capsule, and sometimes they need to be much stiffer and tougher. The joints between your teeth and the sockets in which your teeth rest, for example, do not need much in the way of movement but do need to be strong. Similarly, at the bottom end of the bones in your lower leg the joint between your tibia and fibula doesn't need any movement. That too is a fibrous joint. Fibrous joints allow no appreciable movement and the bones are fixed together by fibrous tissue.

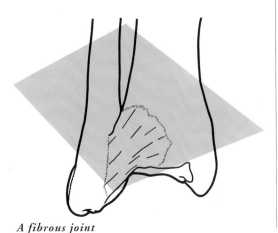

*A fibrous joint*

## CARTILAGINOUS JOINTS

These joints could be described as a halfway house between the synovial joints and the fibrous joints in that they do allow a small amount of movement and they are very strong. The bones of your spine – known as the intervertebral bones – are separated by intervertebral discs which act as shock absorbers. The amount of movement possible between two intervertebral bones is only very small but, when they are added together, all the disc-bone joints give your spine a considerable amount of movement without losing much strength.

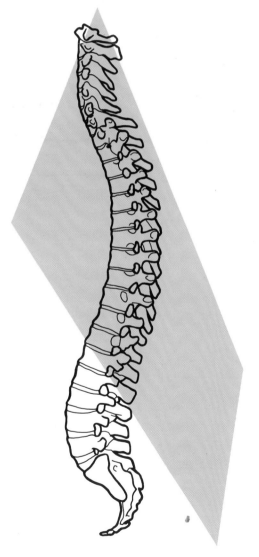

*A cartilaginous joint*

11

## YOUR KNEES AND ELBOWS: SYNOVIAL HINGE JOINTS

Joints which only allow one main type of movement are called 'hinge joints' because they are like hinges! There may, in addition, be some rotational movement as well but this is not a property of the hinge joint itself. (See below).

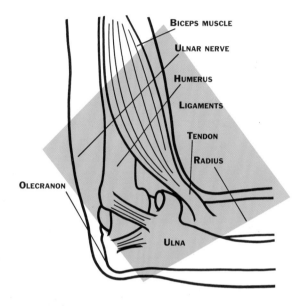

*The elbow is a hinge joint*

## YOUR KNEES

Each knee joint connects two of the strongest long bones in your body – the femur and the tibia. Although the articular surfaces of these two bones do not fit particularly well together the ligaments and muscles around the knee are very strong and make the joint extremely stable. The patella is a small, triangular, flat bone which sits inside the tendon belonging to the quadriceps muscle of the thigh and has two main functions: it minimizes the amount of friction between the quadriceps tendon and the lower end of the femur and it provides the front of the knee with some protection from head-on injury. The patella is not particularly important and if it is damaged it can be removed without affecting the knee very much at all.

## YOUR ELBOWS

Each elbow joint connects the two bones of the forearm – the radius and the ulna – with the humerus, the bone of the upper arm. Your ability to turn your hand over (so that it is either palm upwards or palm downwards) is due to the existence of joints between the radius and the ulna bones in the forearm.

## YOUR SHOULDERS AND HIPS: BALL AND SOCKET JOINTS

Joints which allow a wide range of movement are called 'ball and socket' joints because the end of one bone, which is shaped like a ball, fits into the end of the other.

### YOUR SHOULDERS

Your shoulders are the most mobile joints in your body. The head of the humerus is ball-shaped and it fits into a cavity in the scapula bone. The cavity in the scapula is shallow and it is this shallowness which gives the shoulder joint its exceptional mobility.

### YOUR HIPS

The femur is similar in shape to the humerus but it is bigger and stronger and the ball of bone on its upper end has a neck – usually about 2 inches (5 cm) long – which enables the ball to fit snugly inside the acetabulum (a deep cup-like cavity) of the hip bone.

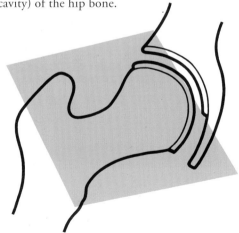

*Ball and socket joints are very mobile*

# YOUR SPINE: A SERIES OF CARTILAGINOUS JOINTS

Your spine is strong enough to withstand pressures of several hundred pounds and is so flexible that it can be bent to form two thirds of a circle. However, the intricate system of muscles, tendons and ligaments which keeps the whole thing together can easily be damaged or disrupted in all sorts of ways. The spine acts as a scaffolding for the whole of the body with the skull, ribs, pelvis and limbs all attached to it. Through its middle runs the extremely delicate spinal cord – so delicate that even a relatively slight physical abnormality can cause severe pain to the victim.

Your spine consists of 26 solid bones, and it is these which give the back its strength. However, if your spine consisted only of solid bone you wouldn't be able to bend down far enough to tie up your shoe laces or to pick things up off the floor, so between the bones there are 23 intervertebral discs which act as bendy shock absorbers.

In addition to giving your spine the strength it needs to support your body the vertebrae also provide essential protection for your spinal cord – your body's biggest nerve. The spinal cord carries impulses from the brain to the arms, legs and body and then carries messages back from those areas to keep the brain informed. Hundreds of individual nerves connect the spinal cord to the various parts of the human body. If your spinal cord is damaged then you will be paralysed, the precise nature of the paralysis depending on the part of the cord that has suffered damage.

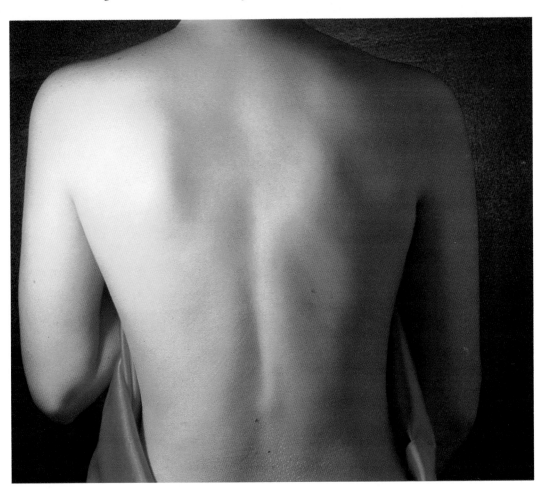

## THE BONES OF YOUR SPINE

The top part of your spine – the neck region – consists of seven bones called the cervical vertebrae. Below them – making up the spinal framework for the chest – are 12 bones known as the thoracic vertebrae.

Next, there are the 5 bones of the lower back – called the lumbar vertebrae.

The sacrum (which although it consists of 5 sacral vertebrae is usually regarded as one bone, since the 5 vertebrae are fixed or fused together) comes next, and right at the bottom there are the 4 tiny vertebrae of the coccyx. Since these are usually joined together, they are often regarded as one bone.

Altogether, then, the spine consists of a grand total of 33 bones. But because five of these bones are joined together to form the sacrum and another four are joined together to form the coccyx, anatomists usually regard the spine as consisting of 26 bones.

The bones at the top and the bottom of the spine – the cervical vertebrae and the bones of the coccyx – are the smallest. The largest bones in the spine are the ones which make up the sacrum and the bones of the lumbar region.

When people draw skeletons – with all the bones of the spine balanced one on top of the other – they usually draw the spine as being fairly straight.

But it isn't straight.

In fact, in order to help it cope with all the stresses and strains of normal everyday life, your spine has no less than four curves. Right at the very top of the spine the small bones of the neck (which are called the cervical vertebrae) curve forwards. Below this curve the thoracic vertebrae – the bones which make up the spine in the chest region – curve backwards. Next, there is the lumbar spine which curves forwards again. And finally, there are the sacrum and the coccyx, which curve backwards.

The bones in your spine differ in size, but despite that they do show a number of similarities. The back part of each vertebra,

called the neural arch, is the most complicated part of each bone. There is a hole through the middle of each neural arch. The spinal cord runs through the holes in all the neural arches. There are several pieces of bone sticking out from the neural arch:

**1. From the back of each neural arch spinous processes stick out. These are the bony projections that you can feel if you touch your spine.**
**2. A bony projection called an 'inferior articular process' points down.**
**3. A bony projection called a 'superior articular process' points up.**
**4. From each side of every neural arch a 'transverse process' projects.**
**5. There is a solid piece of bone called the 'body' at the front of each vertebra.**

## THE JOINTS IN THE SPINE

Amazingly, the bones in the spine are joined together by a total of nearly 150 joints. Every single one of these joints helps to hold the spinal bones together firmly to create the apparently 'solid' spine. It is these 150 joints that make your spine strong.

Arthritis can affect any of these joints and so the possibilities for pain and stiffness in the spine are clearly tremendous.

Every one of the 26 vertebrae that make up the spine is connected to the vertebra above it and the vertebra below it. At the very bottom of the spine, the sacrum – made up of the sacral bones – is joined to the hip bones. At the top of the spine the skull rests on the first cervical vertebra. The thoracic vertebrae help to provide a solid foundation for the twelve ribs which protect the heart and lungs and form the foundation of the chest wall.

## THE DISCS BETWEEN THE BONES

Unless your spine is really badly affected by arthritis it will still be bendable. And a perfectly healthy spine is amazing – it can be bent round in a quite remarkable way.

Clearly, if the spine consisted solely of bone this would be impossible. A solid spine – consisting of vertebrae fixed together – would not bend. It is the shape of the bones and the existence of the disks in between the bones which make the bending of the spine possible.

The intervertebral disks, which fit in between the individual vertebrae and which are known as the spine's shock absorbers, help to make sure that your spine can bend and move in all sorts of different directions without a terrible crunching of bone on bone.

On the outside of each intervertebral disk there is a strong, fibrous case which is called the annular fibrosus. Inside that there is a soft, very squashy interior called the nucleus pulposus. The nucleus pulposus is strengthened with fibre.

The disks are particularly squashy because they are made up mainly of fluid – they have no blood and a very rudimentary nerve supply.

At night when you lie down in bed the intervertebral disks in your spine expand and get larger as they fill up with food and with water. During the day, however, as you walk about, the vertebrae will compress the disks in between them and some of the fluid will be squeezed out. Because of this squeezing and compressing, we tend to lose around half an inch (1.3 cm) in height during the daytime. At night, when our disks expand again, we regain our lost height.

Although the intervertebral disks play the most important part in giving the spine its movement, the shape of the vertebrae themselves also has a part to play. For example, the first cervical vertebra allows your head to tilt sideways and to nod forwards and backwards; the second cervical vertebra allows your head to turn to the right and to the left; and the other bones in the spine also allow you to move your spine a little.

## THE LIGAMENTS

The 150 joints which help to make up the spine are protected and given added strength by the protection of a huge number of ligaments; strong, fibrous and slightly elastic bands of tissue which hold the two pieces of bone together wherever a joint is formed. Because of the way the fibres which make up a ligament run, the ligaments help to ensure that each joint is held firmly and is able to move properly.

## CAN JOINTS BE MADE MORE FLEXIBLE?

The range of movement in any particular joint depends upon the shape of the bones, the design of the joint and the restricting actions of ligaments and muscles. You cannot do anything about the design of the joint (in other words you can't turn a 'hinge' joint into a 'ball and socket' joint) and you can't deliberately alter the shape of the bones in a particular joint but, by training, you can modify the restraining action of the ligaments and muscles which control the amount of movement in a joint. Professional acrobats, gymnasts and dancers achieve a tremendous amount of flexibility in their joints, but they usually start their training very early in life and they always train hard for long periods.

## WHY ARE SOME PEOPLE DOUBLE-JOINTED?

Individuals who have an unusual amount of movement in a joint are often described as 'double-jointed'. 'Double joints' are common in the joints of the hand. The implication is that the extra amount of movement is brought about by two joints or one unusually shaped joint. In fact, this is not true – people who seem to be double-jointed are usually merely able to dislocate a particular joint. There is usually an audible click as this happens.

## WHY DO SOME JOINTS MAKE A NOISE?

The clicking of joints can be caused by tendons or ligaments that slip, by joints dislocating or even by small bubbles of gas moving about. When a joint makes a grating noise it is usually because the cartilage has worn down and the underlying bones are rubbing on one another.

# CHAPTER TWO

# Rheumatoid Arthritis

*There is little doubt that rheumatoid arthritis is one of the commonest of all crippling long-term diseases. Although it usually affects the smaller joints – particularly those of the hands, wrists and feet – it can also attack the joints of the spine. However, the spine is usually the last part of the body to be affected. The neck is usually the first part of the spine to succumb.*

## THE SYMPTOMS OF RHEUMATOID ARTHRITIS

The initial symptoms of rheumatoid arthritis are usually pain, tenderness, swelling and stiffness of the joints that are affected. These symptoms, which can arrive quite suddenly or develop slowly over a lengthy period of time, are nearly always worst first thing in the morning. Many joints can be implicated and sufferers who have rheumatoid arthritis badly may complain that their whole body is affected. The pain and aching is often accompanied by a general feeling of tiredness, listlessness and of being run down.

The symptoms of rheumatoid arthritis are unusual in that they may sometimes disappear almost completely without any warning – though, sadly, they usually come back again.

## WHAT ARE THE CAUSES OF RHEUMATOID ARTHRITIS?

There is no known single cause of rheumatoid arthritis. Instead, it seems likely that a number of different factors may be responsible for its development.

### 1. Infection

It is possible that the development of the disease may be triggered by a virus (see auto-immune reaction, below).

### 2. Inherited factors

Some genes transmitted from generation to generation seem to determine susceptibility to rheumatoid arthritis (i.e. whether or not you get it) while others determine the extent to which the disease develops (i.e. how badly you get it).

### 3. Food

It seems possible that certain types of food may make rheumatoid arthritis more likely. Meat – and meat products – may be a cause of rheumatoid arthritis. On page 82 you will find dietary advice to follow in order to reduce your chances of getting rheumatoid arthritis and minimize your symptoms if you have already got it.

### 4. Auto-immune reaction

Normally, your immune system helps to protect you against attack from infectious diseases. However, because the changes which take place inside the joints when rheumatoid arthritis develops are similar to the changes which take place in other parts of the body when antibodies produced by the body are fighting an infection, many experts now believe that under some circumstances the body's immune system may be triggered to attack the joints (and in particular the lining of the joints), producing an inflammation of the synovial membrane which causes the well-known symptoms of the disease. One of the blood tests commonly done to confirm the presence of rheumatoid arthritis in joints checks for a special protein in the bloodstream. This protein is an antibody – similar to the antibodies the body produces when it overcomes an infection such as influenza or measles. No one really understands yet exactly how or why the body's immune defence system should attack the

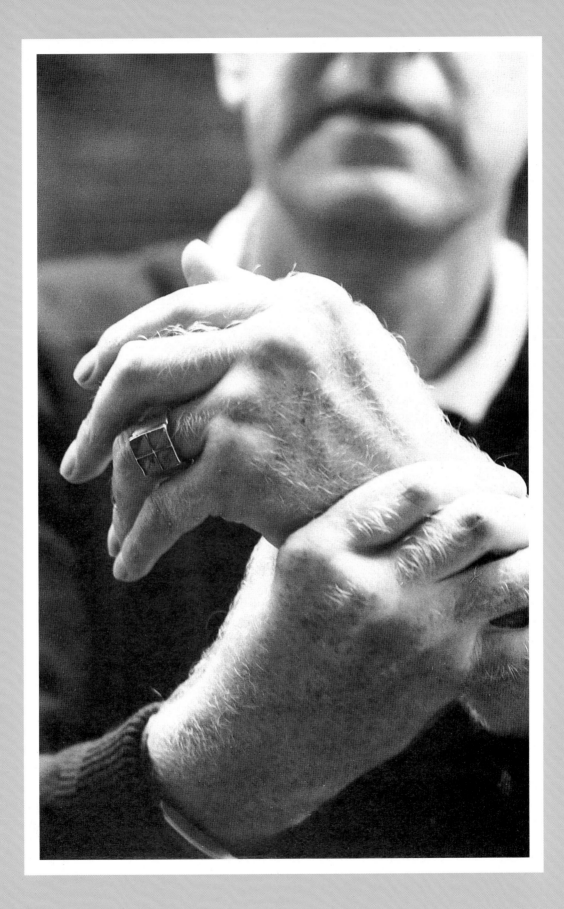

linings of the joints, but it may be nothing more complicated than a simple case of mistaken identity. Normally, cells called macrophages travel around the body looking for foreign cells. If they find any they immediately produce a chemical signal which calls for help. Within a short space of time the foreign cells will be surrounded by cells called 'killer lymphocytes' which either poison them to death or eat them alive. This is, in principle, how the immune defence system of your body functions.

Normally, neither the macrophages nor the 'killer lymphocytes' are triggered into action by the body's own cells. However, if any of the latter have become damaged and have lost their identifying marks the 'killer lymphocytes' will deal with them just as effectively and as unsympathetically as they will deal with hostile foreign viruses, bacteria or fungi.

In rheumatoid arthritis your macrophages and 'killer lymphocytes' may be triggered into action by the fact that certain cells in your body –

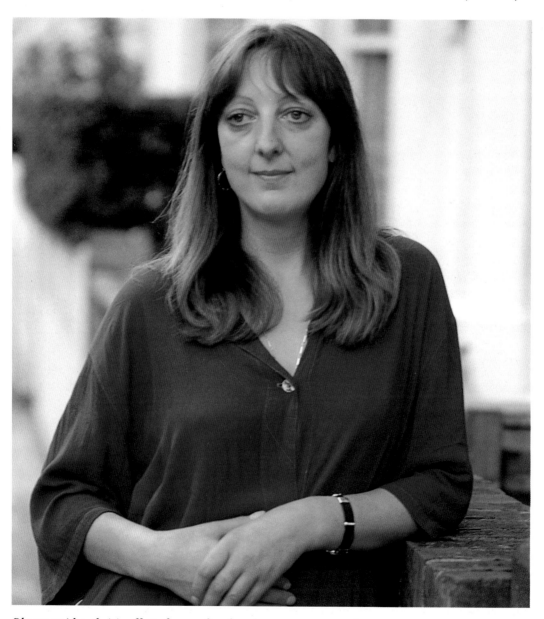

*Rheumatoid arthritis affects four or five females to every two males.*

notably the cells of the synovial membranes in your joints – have changed in some way which is not as yet understood. It is thought that this is where a virus may come into play, for it is possible that a virus may change your synovial membrane in some slight way so that it appears to be 'foreign' to your defensive macrophages and 'killer lymphocytes'.

## WHO GETS RHEUMATOID ARTHRITIS?

Rheumatoid arthritis is much commoner in women than in men – for every two males who get the disease there are usually four or five female sufferers. This difference may be due to some genetic factor carried on the female sex chromosomes. Rheumatoid arthritis also runs in families and if your parents, grandparents or brothers or sisters have or had the disease your chances of suffering from it are increased. Although the disease can appear at any age it most commonly starts in early adulthood or early middle age. Rheumatoid arthritis has been found in countries all over the world and it affects members of all races but it is more common – and tends to be more severe – among the inhabitants of Northern Europe. No one really knows whether this is due to the climate, to genetic factors or to a localized infection.

## HOW COMMON IS RHEUMATOID ARTHRITIS?

It is difficult to say how common the disease is because not all sufferers seek medical help. Obviously, some patients have far more severe symptoms and they will nearly all visit their doctor for advice. However, patients with mild symptoms are likely to struggle on without seeing a doctor. Some will manage without any treatment at all while others will treat themselves or visit alternative medical practitioners. Severe rheumatoid arthritis probably affects about one in every 200 people (with an even smaller percentage being affected so acutely that they become crippled), whereas mild rheumatoid arthritis probably affects about one in every 50 people.

## WHAT HAPPENS TO THE JOINTS IN RHEUMATOID ARTHRITIS?

The normal job of the synovium – the membrane which covers the joint – is to produce a constant supply of synovial fluid, the oily substance which lubricates, moistens and feeds the cartilage on the ends of the two opposing bones. It is the cartilages which take all the pressure when a joint is in action and it is the synovial fluid which ensures that the cartilages stay in good condition.

When rheumatoid arthritis develops and the synovial membrane becomes inflamed the first thing that happens is that the membrane swells up as the blood vessels supplying it open up to bring more 'killer' blood cells into the area.

If you have an infected spot on your skin, the blood vessels supplying that area will open up in an attempt to take more white blood cells to the area to help tackle the infection. Your body's internal defence systems rely on your blood supply to get to trouble spots and wherever there is a problem the localized blood vessels open up to ensure that the local blood supply is increased to the absolute maximum.

This is exactly what happens to the synovium in an inflamed joint that is affected by rheumatoid arthritis. Your body assumes that there must be some external agent present (a bacteria, virus or some other foreign organism) to cause the inflammation and so it sends teams of specialist 'killer' blood cells to the area to try to clear up the problem. In addition to becoming swollen, the synovium also starts to go red and to feel hot as the blood flow increases.

Because the synovium gets its nourishment from its blood supply the increased flow means that it starts to over-produce synovial fluid and within a relatively short time the whole joint will become swollen with fluid and painful to touch or to move. Instead of making movement easier, the extra synovial fluid makes it more difficult than ever. Occasionally, particularly in the knee joint, the excess fluid inside the joint can build up such a high pressure that it bursts the joint capsule and escapes into the muscles of the calf.

The joint will by now be showing all the typical symptoms of rheumatoid arthritis: it will be swollen, it will feel hot to the touch, it will look red and it will be stiff and painful to move.

Meanwhile, because the inflammation is still there, your body assumes that the underlying infection, which it wrongly believes has caused the inflammation, is simply proving too powerful and too resistant to the 'killer' cells in your blood supply. So your body responds aggressively by increasing the flow of blood still further – pumping ever-increasing amounts of blood into the tissues and making things worse and worse rather than better. The inevitable result of this is that the synovium just gets bigger and bigger, gradually spreading over more and more of the inside of the joint.

Eventually, the expanding synovium will start to damage the cartilage – the load-bearing surface on the ends of the opposing bones of the joint. Instead of being slippery and making the joint move easily and smoothly, the cartilage will become rough and pitted, making movement difficult and uncomfortable. In advanced rheumatoid arthritis the joints which are affected will become deformed as well as swollen and stiff.

If the tendons and bursae which lie over the joint are also affected by the inflammation, they will be damaged in much the same way, and the area around the joint will become tender to the touch and difficult to move.

One of the tragedies of rheumatoid arthritis is undoubtedly the fact that the problems which develop are caused by the body's own defence mechanisms mistakenly diagnosing a case of mild inflammation as being caused by an underlying infection; they then overreact and pump unwanted blood cells into the area in such huge quantities that the joint becomes permanently

*"Patients who suffer from rheumatoid arthritis often complain that they feel tired, easily exhausted, irritable and edgy."*

diseased. It is, I suppose, rather like the fire brigade turning out to a small fire and then causing far more damage with their high-pressure water hoses than has been caused by the flames.

Normally, inflammation is a useful trigger. It encourages your body's own defence mechanisms to act quickly and decisively, limiting the amount of damage, getting rid of the cause of the inflammation and encouraging the healing process. As soon as it is clear that the underlying cause of the inflammation has been dealt with, your body will stop sending in 'killer' blood cells.

However, in rheumatoid arthritis the inflammation doesn't go away and it is your body's reaction rather than the inflammation itself that does most of the damage. The consequences can be long-lasting and, if untreated, permanently disabling.

## RHEUMATOID ARTHRITIS DOES NOT JUST AFFECT YOUR JOINTS

If you suffer from rheumatoid arthritis it will not only be your joints which will be affected. Because the inflammation inside your joint (or joints) triggers an auto-immune reaction and inspires your body to send an increased blood supply into the joints which are involved, the disease will affect your health in many other ways.

Patients who suffer from rheumatoid arthritis often complain that they feel tired, easily exhausted, irritable and edgy. Most victims claim that they also have vague aches and pains in many different parts of their bodies. It is quite common for rheumatoid arthritis sufferers to complain that they constantly feel as though they have the 'flu. Many have night sweats and quite a few find that they lose weight (though this can be an advantage for it can help reduce the severity of the symptoms associated with arthritis – see page 82).

Many people with rheumatoid arthritis show a slight rise in body temperature, partly because of the increased blood flow and partly because your body knows that one of the best ways to combat an infection (which it thinks you have) is by increasing your general body temperature.

And because the blood system is concentrating on producing and disseminating 'killer' blood cells there may be a shortage of red cells – the sort that normally carry oxygen to the tissues. This shortage of red blood cells can lead to anaemia and to breathlessness and tiredness.

Finally, although it is usually the joints – and particularly the synovial membranes – which are affected by the inflammation associated with rheumatoid arthritis, that same inflammation can sometimes affect other parts of the body. The skin, kidneys, eyes, nerves, heart, lungs and tendons can all be affected by inflammation occasionally, and when this happens all sorts of other symptoms can develop. Bones may become thin and easily broken, lungs may be scarred and the skin may be ulcerated.

## HOW QUICKLY DOES RHEUMATOID ARTHRITIS DEVELOP?

Very occasionally rheumatoid arthritis will start suddenly. It is possible for someone to go to bed feeling perfectly healthy and to wake up the next morning with all the symptoms of rheumatoid arthritis in one or more joints. However, it is much more common for it to develop slowly over a period of weeks or even months.

The disease usually starts in the joints of either the hands or the feet. In a typical patient the joints of the fingers will become stiff and swollen and painful to move (the stiffness is usually worst first thing in the morning). Because it hurts to move the joints the patient will probably want to rest them as much as possible. And so the muscles will become weak and will start to shrink.

Gradually, as the pain and stiffness in the small joints get worse, so the generalized symptoms of tiredness and weakness will also develop.

## WHICH JOINTS ARE AFFECTED?

Any joint in the body that contains a synovial membrane can develop rheumatoid arthritis. The small joints of the hands and feet are the ones most commonly affected to begin with – the joints in the middle and base of the fingers are probably the ones which are affected most frequently. Next are usually the wrists and the knees. The ankles, elbows, shoulders and hips are affected less frequently.

## RHEUMATOID ARTHRITIS CAN LAST A LONG TIME

The bad news is that once rheumatoid arthritis has started to develop it will usually last for many years before finally burning itself out and ceasing to cause any more damage. However, the good news is that the disease comes and goes and most sufferers notice that their symptoms quieten down after a year or two – although they may flare up occasionally.

During an active phase of the disease patients usually feel very ill and invariably wake up feeling stiff. Joints which are affected have to be loosened slowly and painfully and they often become stiff and painful again in the late afternoon or early evening. Most sufferers who have active rheumatoid arthritis have to do things slowly.

Some patients have noticed that active phases can be triggered by certain types of food or by doing too much. Others find it quite impossible to spot any factor as being responsible for a painful attack.

During an active phase the inflamed synovium usually does damage to the inside of the joint and so, afterwards, the amount of movement in the joint will probably be slightly reduced. The hands, which have small and apparently vulnerable joints, seem to suffer most and to show the most dramatic long-term changes.

After a few years rheumatoid arthritis usually begins to settle down and the active phases become less and less common. In some patients this settling down occurs after just a year or two.

In others it can take 20 or 30 years. Even if your arthritis has been active for many, many years you should never give up hope that it will one day become inactive, although your joints may have been permanently damaged and disfigured by that time.

The joints of the hands – which often show the worst distortion and which may be so badly damaged that fine movements are difficult or even completely impossible – are usually least painful in the chronic or non-active stages of the disease. In contrast, the joints of the hips and knees – which have to carry a lot of weight – may not show a great deal of deformity but may be constantly painful.

## TENDONS CAN BE AFFECTED TOO

Although rheumatoid arthritis is primarily a joint disease it can sometimes affect the thin, cord-like tendons by which muscles are attached to the bones which make up a joint. When a muscle contracts the tendon is used to pull the bone into place. Inevitably, the pressure on and in the tendon can be very high.

Tendons can be affected in two ways.

First, the tendons themselves may develop patches of inflammation. When this happens a lump or nodule may develop inside or on top of the tendon. Normally, tendons slide in and out of place quite smoothly and easily – often travelling through fairly close-fitting tunnels so that they do not interfere with (or get troubled by) other tissues. However, when a nodule develops on a tendon the tendon may have difficulty in sliding in and out of its tunnel. To begin with it may move in and out of position with an audible 'click'. For a while it may be possible to force the lumpy tendon through its tunnel but if the lump gets big enough the tendon will stick permanently in one position.

Second, because the narrow tissue tunnels through which many tendons pass are lined with exactly the same sort of synovial membrane as that which lines and lubricates the inside of the

joint, the inflammation of rheumatoid arthritis may cause the inside of the tunnel to become swollen. The result will be that the tunnel becomes narrower and stickier – and so, not surprisingly, the tendon will tend to stick in one position. If the tendon remains stuck for long enough, there is a real danger that the inflamed synovial membrane will start to 'eat' it in just the same way that the inflamed synovial membrane inside a joint will eat into the cartilage surfaces on the tops of the bones. Eventually, there is a danger that the tendon will become weak and may tear apart, with the result that the muscle is no longer connected to the bone that it is supposed to move. Inevitably, the result is then a paralysis. Putting a joint in a splint can sometimes help encourage the torn tendon to heal itself and if that fails it is often possible to repair a tendon surgically by simply sewing together the two separated halves.

## THE NEED TO REMAIN ACTIVE

Because of the damage done inside the joints that are affected, patients with rheumatoid arthritis sometimes become disabled. If the hands are badly affected by damaged joints or displaced or torn tendons all the fingers may bend to one side or individual fingers may bend in a variety of different directions, making it difficult to use the hand. If the toes are badly affected walking may be made difficult. Patients who have bad arthritis in their feet complain that walking – even in comfortable shoes – is like walking on a stony beach in bare feet. If the toes become displaced in the same way that fingers often are the foot probably won't fit into a normal shoe.

If the elbows are badly affected the sufferer may have difficulty in bending or straightening his or her arm. This can make all sorts of things – from washing to eating to tooth-cleaning – extremely difficult. If the knees or hips are badly deformed the sufferer will find that walking can be very difficult.

## JOINT DAMAGE MAY RESULT IN DISABLEMENT

Not surprisingly, the constant pain and disablement caused by rheumatoid arthritis often make sufferers very depressed. They may find it difficult to remain active, and it can seem easier to stay at home slumped in an easy chair than to go out with friends or pursue hobbies.

But staying slumped in a chair or in bed can produce extra problems.

First, there are the physical hazards. Staying immobile for long periods can result in muscles becoming weaker than ever and bones becoming thinner and more likely to break. Areas of skin which support the body can develop pressure sores. Sitting or lying down for long periods means that the consumption of calories goes down – and since most people who spend long periods sitting or lying eat too much that means a potentially dangerous and destructive weight gain. Infections are far more likely in people

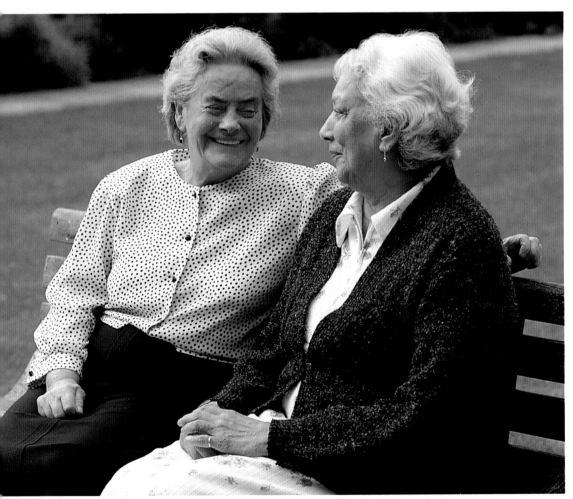

*It is important not to let rheumatoid arthritis prevent you from going out and about.*

who don't move about and, of course, the joints are more likely to get so stiff that movement becomes quite impossible. Finally, people who spend a lot of time keeping still tend to become less tolerant of pain when it occurs. And thus a vicious circle develops.

Second, there are the mental hazards. If you allow your rheumatoid arthritis to run your whole life you will quickly become demoralized and miserable. Boredom, anxiety and fear quickly lead to an increased susceptibility to stress and a far greater liability to depression.

## WHAT TESTS CAN BE DONE FOR RHEUMATOID ARTHRITIS?

Because rheumatoid arthritis is common and because the symptoms are pretty obvious it isn't usually difficult to make the diagnosis clinically, without any hospital or laboratory tests.

However, diagnosis is not always easy, particularly in the early stages of the disease.

**• Blood tests may show the existence of a substance called 'the rheumatoid factor' and may show that there is inflammation in the body. They can usually provide useful results early on in the history of the disease.**

**• X-rays may show that the edges of the bones are damaged – but abnormalities are not usually noticeable until the rheumatoid arthritis has been present for many months or even years.**

**• Testing the synovial fluid – taken out of the joint – may show the presence of the disease. Repeated tests may enable doctors to tell how fast the disease is progressing.**

## CAN RHEUMATOID ARTHRITIS BE TREATED?

Rheumatoid arthritis cannot be cured but it can be treated and it is much easier to prevent complications developing than it is to treat them once they have developed. Never forget that although you may become disabled as a result of having rheumatoid arthritis it is extremely unlikely to kill you.

## THE RIGHT ATTITUDE IS VITAL

If you approach your arthritis gloomily – anxious about possible disablement and depressed by the fact that there is no 'magic' cure available – the disease will do you far more damage than if you approach the problem in a positive, even aggressive, frame of mind. Reading this book will help you enormously because the more you know about the disease the greater your chance of combating it successfully. There are many things that your doctor can do to help you, but there are also many things that you can do to help yourself – and approaching your disease in a positive frame of mind is one of the most important ways to begin.

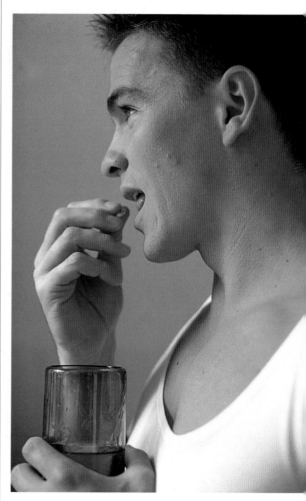

*Aspirin, one of the most well-known painkillers, is very effective for arthritic pain.*

# What Can Doctors Do to Help Combat Rheumatoid Arthritis?

## Drug Therapy

There are scores of drugs for the treatment of arthritis – in all its forms – and the number available is growing every month. Many patients with rheumatoid arthritis need to keep taking medication for months or even years and that means that there are huge potential profits to be made by companies which can develop and market safe and effective drugs. It is hardly surprising, therefore, that most of the major international drug companies produce at least one drug designed for the relief of joint symptoms such as pain and stiffness.

## Aspirin and Co: The Non-Steroidal Anti-Inflammatory Drugs

The 'non-steroidal anti-inflammatory drugs' are the ones most commonly prescribed. Drugs in this category work in three different ways:
- **They reduce inflammation**
- **They help conquer pain**
- **They reduce any fever that may be present.**

Selecting the right drug for the right patient is always something of a problem; some patients will respond to one drug while others will react best to another. It is often a question of trial and error before the right drug is found.

Surprisingly, perhaps, the drug that is still most widely prescribed – and which still seems to offer the greatest number of patients the greatest amount of relief – is aspirin, the first 'non-steroidal anti-inflammatory drug'. Aspirin has an unfortunate reputation for causing stomach bleeding but when used properly and carefully and prescribed in the soluble form it is as safe as most of the competing products. During the last decade or so an enormous number of 'safe' alternatives have been produced but time and time again it has been shown that the newer drugs will also produce similar symptoms if used in reasonable quantities or for fairly long periods. The main disadvantage with aspirin is that it needs to be taken regularly and patients using it invariably have to take tablets every four hours or so. Some patients do develop allergies to aspirin and occasionally tinnitus (noises in the ears) and deafness can also be a problem.

Because aspirin is made by numerous companies and sold at very competitive prices most drug companies prefer to manufacture and promote their own alternatives – which can be sold at a much higher price and which can, therefore, be far more profitable. Consequently, there are scores of alternatives which have roughly similar properties. It is impossible to recommend any one of these drugs as being better than any other and new drugs are launched virtually every month. Although there are many chemical differences between the drugs, the majority work by relieving both pain and inflammation. Most doctors have their own favourite drugs with which they become familiar, though some do tend to prescribe the latest (and probably the most expensive) product that the drug salesmen tell them about. The only advantage of the huge variety of 'non-steroidal anti-inflammatory drugs' (known as NSAIDS) is that if you fail to get relief from one drug there will almost always be another drug for you to try.

## Corticosteroids

Corticosteroids (also known as 'steroids') suppress inflammation so effectively that when they were first introduced they were hailed as 'miracle' drugs. They mimic the actions of corticosteroid hormones produced within the body as an internal anti-inflammatory. Unfortunately, although (or perhaps that should be 'because') they are very powerful corticosteroids can cause very serious side-effects. They can produce stomach troubles, blood pressure problems, bone disorders, skin diseases and a characteristic swelling of the face and body. There is also a danger that if you take a corticosteroid for too long your body's own production of steroids will shut down and you will become dependent on the tablets you are taking.

## GETTING THE BEST OUT OF MEDICINES

Sadly, many doctors do not really understand exactly how drugs work and what they can and cannot do. However, if you are going to benefit properly from the drugs you are prescribed, it is vitally important that you understand just how drugs work and what you can expect from them.

One survey which was done recently showed that a majority of patients – and this includes patients who are at home and patients receiving in-patient hospital attention – receive only one quarter of the dose of pain killer they need in order to provide them with proper relief!

This is not, of course, because doctors or nurses are mean-spirited or uncaring. There are several reasons for the medical profession's failure to give patients enough pain killers.

First, it is very easy for both doctors and nurses to underestimate the amount of pain a patient is suffering. Lots of patients try to be brave and not show just how much pain they are in. Inevitably, therefore, when doctors prescribe pills they don't prescribe large enough doses.

Secondly, both doctors and nurses worry a lot about their patients getting hooked on the drugs they are taking. They worry about this because some pain killers – and in particular the morphine derivatives – are addictive. In fact, this fear is to a very large extent unfounded. It is very rare for patients to get hooked on pain killers – even if they need to take quite large doses for long periods of time. Indeed, the risk of addiction seems to be greater if a patient does not receive his drug often enough or in adequate

## WHAT YOU SHOULD KNOW ABOUT DRUGS

**1. HOW MANY TIMES A DAY SHOULD THEY BE TAKEN? If a drug has to be taken once a day, it doesn't usually matter at what time of day it is taken as long as it is taken at the same time of day. A drug that needs to be taken twice a day should usually be taken at intervals of twelve hours. And a drug that needs to be taken three times a day should usually be taken at eight hour intervals.**

**2. DOES IT MATTER WHETHER THE DRUG IS TAKEN BEFORE, DURING OR AFTER MEALS? Some drugs are not absorbed properly if taken with food – other drugs may cause stomach problems and need to be taken with meals.**

**3. FOR HOW LONG MUST A DRUG BE TAKEN? Some drugs need to be taken as a complete course - others can be stopped when symptoms cease. It is essential that you know which of the drugs you take fall into which of these categories.**

**4. WHAT SIDE EFFECTS CAN YOU EXPECT? You should ask your doctor if there are any particular side effects that you should watch out for. And if you notice any side effects of symptoms while taking a drug you should get in touch with your doctor straight away, report what you have noticed and ask him whether you should keep on with the pills or whether you should stop them. Common side effects with pain relievers include constipation, indigestion, dizziness and nausea and vomiting. But it is important to remember that all drugs can cause side effects and that the range of possible side effects is virtually infinite.**

quantities to control the pain. When a patient has to suffer pain and wait for his drug he is more likely to get hooked on that drug than when the dosage and the timing are designed to enable the patient to avoid or to control the pain.

One of the most important things you should remember is that you will suffer far less if you take your pain killers regularly according to the clock, rather than waiting for the pain to return before taking them.

If you only take your pain killer when your pain is terrible your body will be weakened and you will be learning to link your drug with relief from pain, which could lead to the problem of drug dependence.

Another very important consideration is that of side effects. You should always ask your doctor if there are any particular side effects that you should watch out for, while taking a drug. And if you notice any side effects while taking drugs, you should get in touch with your doctor straight away, report what you have noticed and ask him whether you should keep on with the pills or whether you should stop them. Common side effects with pain relievers include constipation, indigestion, dizziness and nausea and vomiting. But it is important to remember that all drugs can cause side effects and that the range of possibilities is virtually infinite.

My advice is that anyone taking a drug of any kind should talk to his or her doctor about the medication. Find out what the drug is prescribed for; find out whether the drug is likely to be needed as a long term or short term measure; and ask your doctor to explain to you how the drug does its job. If your doctor doesn't know the answers to these questions, then maybe your questions will help to make sure that he does a little homework himself so he is in a position to answer questions in future.

*"Gastritis is the commonest side-effect associated with most of the drugs that are widely used in the treatment of rheumatoid arthritis."*

## SUPPOSITORIES

When you swallow a pill, the active constituent in that pill gets into your bloodstream and therefore the rest of your body by being digested as it travels along the intestinal tract.

As far as the drugs used to control arthritic symptoms are concerned, the main danger with this method is that the walls of the stomach may be irritated by the drug. Gastritis is, indeed, the commonest side-effect associated with most of the drugs that are widely used in the treatment of rheumatoid arthritis.

However, drugs do not have to be given by mouth in order to be absorbed through the digestive system and into the bloodstream. In some countries the other end of the intestinal tract – the rectum – is considered a far more sensible place from which to start the absorption process. A drug taken as a suppository will be absorbed into the body just as quickly as a drug taken in tablet form, but there will be a much reduced chance of any intestinal irritation. Although there may be obvious difficulties for patients with severe rheumatoid arthritis (putting a suppository into your rectum may be tricky if you have deformed, arthritic hands) the advantages are considerable and many drugs are available in this form.

## INJECTIONS

Drugs taken by mouth or in suppository form have to travel throughout the whole body in order to have an effect on painful and inflamed joints. It is often more efficient to put the drug directly into the joint concerned. This means not only that the joint gets the full benefit of the drug but that the patient concerned is spared whatever side-effects may be associated with the drug when it is used generally.

When joints are being injected it is obviously

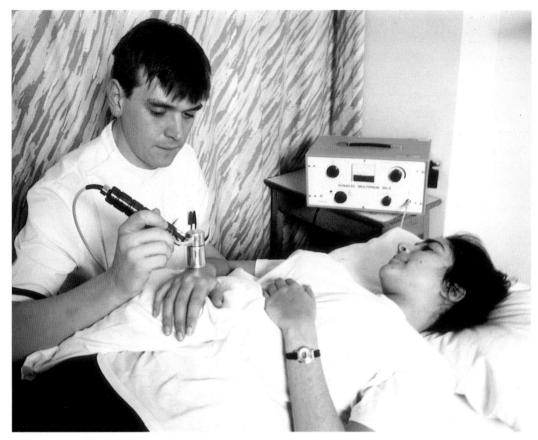

*Physiotherapists use many techniques, including short wave diathermy and interferential therapy.*

important that the person handling the needle knows exactly what he or she is doing. Carelessly or improperly administered injections can do far more harm than good. Some general practitioners do inject straight into joints (these are known as intra-articular injections) but the majority of patients will usually be dealt with by some sort of specialist – normally either an orthopaedic surgeon or a rheumatologist.

The shoulders, wrists, elbows and knees are the joints most commonly injected, although other joints (fingers, toes and hips, for example) can be tackled in this way.

The drug used for the injection is usually a corticosteroid. The risks associated with drugs in this group are much smaller when the drugs are injected directly into a joint than when they are taken by mouth and allowed to spread throughout the whole body.

Before giving an injection into a joint the

doctor will usually clean the area with an antiseptic and then give a local anaesthetic to numb the skin and the tissues just under it. The doctor usually confirms that he has the needle in the right place – right inside the joint – by withdrawing some of the fluid through the needle before giving the injection.

Improvement usually follows about three days after an injection and will last for several months. A steroid injection can be repeated two or three times a year if necessary. Since infection can develop after an intra-articular injection it is important to tell your doctor straight away if you develop any unusual symptoms (such as increased pain, swelling, redness or heat) after the injection.

If a joint is swollen with fluid it may be possible to reduce the amount of pain, swelling and stiffness by withdrawing some of the excess fluid from the joint before giving an injection.

## SURGERY

Although surgery is used fairly frequently in the treatment of patients with osteoarthritis its use is relatively rare in cases of rheumatoid arthritis. However, there are some operations that may be performed in the treatment of this disease. They include the following:

### SYNOVECTOMY

If the joint lining or synovium is badly inflamed it may be possible to prevent damage to the joint by removing the inflamed synovium completely. This operation needs to be performed at an early stage in the progress of the disease, before too much damage has been done. Similarly, if the tunnels through which the tendons pass are affected by an inflamed synovium an operation to remove the damaged tunnel may prevent problems in the future. Again, this is usually done at an early stage of the disease to prevent severe disabling.

### JOINT REPLACEMENT

Joint replacement operations were originally devised for use on patients with osteoarthritis where large joints, such as the hip, are commonly affected. Large joint operations have been so successful (nine out of ten operations on patients who need hip replacements are effective) that surgeons are now replacing knee, elbow, shoulder, ankle and finger joints.

### NERVE RELIEF

If a nerve is trapped by inflamed or swollen tissues the numbness, continuous pain and 'pins and needles' that are produced can be excruciating to the patient. An operation to free the nerve and remove the pressure can produce spectacularly successful results.

## PHYSIOTHERAPY

A good physiotherapist will probably want to see you walk and sit and move before he or she even begins to examine you. By watching the way that you move, the physiotherapist will be able to tell a great deal about your arthritis, the state of your joints and the extent of your pain.

Then, when he has studied your movements, he or she will want to examine you.

Physiotherapists don't just use their hands to heal their patients – they also use them to find out what is wrong. By moving your joints and by feeling your muscles, a physiotherapist will be able to measure the extent of the damage done by your arthritis and will be able to work out how best he or she can help you.

In addition to watching their patients move and examining them with their hands, many physiotherapists also like to look at any X-rays that may have been taken – or, at the very least, to look at the X-ray reports written by the radiologist. In addition, they will also want to look at any blood tests which may have been done.

Once they have thoroughly researched the patient's condition, physiotherapists can start with their treatment. Unlike drugs, which are often designed to offer nothing more than short-term relief, physiotherapy is usually designed to provide some form of long-term improvement.

The type of treatments physiotherapists use varies a great deal, of course, but their repertoire includes massage, manipulation and exercise.

**The sort of manipulation techniques used by physiotherapists are rather similar to the ones used by chiropractors and osteopaths. It is vitally important that joints and bones which are damaged are never manipulated (and it is especially important that a damaged spine is never manipulated in any way. If it were, there would be a risk of causing permanent damage to the spinal cord). It is also unwise to allow anyone to manipulate an inflamed joint or a bone which is weakened (this means that many patients with arthritis will probably not be suitable for manipulation). When the joints and bones are suitable for manipulation the operator will often be able to unlock joints that have become fixed simply by using his or her hands. When properly used, manipulation can help to relieve joint stiffness and muscle spasm.**

**A professional masseur (or masseuse) will stroke, knead and stretch your skin and mus-**

cles in order to relax them and to help take the stress and strain out of your joints. A good massage will help to break up toughened tissues and may even be able to help improve a poor blood supply. You can, of course, have a massage from a friend, but a professional masseur is likely to be able to help relieve pains and stiffness far more effectively. As with manipulation you should not allow anyone to massage you unless your doctor has given his or her approval.

## ULTRASOUND

Because it shows up soft tissues which cannot be shown very well on X-ray pictures, doctors use ultrasound to help them make a diagnosis. Physiotherapists, on the other hand, use ultrasound, which consists of high frequency sound waves, as a treatment aid to help them to mend injured ligaments, joints and muscles. Ultrasound is believed to help in several ways: it speeds up the ordinary, natural healing process; it increases the blood flow in the area and it also reduces the amount of inflammation.

## TRANSCUTANEOUS NERVE STIMULATION

Devices called TENS machines can be very effective in controlling pain. How they work is described on page 68.

## SHORT WAVE DIATHERMY

Like ultrasound, a full course of short wave diathermy is likely to involve two or three sessions a week for several weeks. And as with ultrasound, those who use this technique, which employs high frequency electromagnetic waves which create heat within the tissues, claim that there are few, if any, significant side effects and that it is painless.

Physiotherapists use short wave diathermy because they claim that it can help to increase the flow of the blood, speed up the healing processes which normally and naturally help to repair the body and reduce any swelling which exists. The precise type of treatment they use will depend upon the tissues involved, for different types of treatment affect tissues at different layers.

## WHAT CAN YOU DO TO HELP OVERCOME RHEUMATOID ARTHRITIS?

### 1. LOSE ANY UNNECESSARY WEIGHT
Every pound of excess weight that you carry around with you puts an additional strain on all your joints, will make existing rheumatoid arthritis worse and will weaken otherwise healthy joints. Advice on how to lose unnecessary weight permanently is given on pages 50–59.

### 2. GIVE UP MEAT
A vegetarian diet is more healthy if you are a sufferer from rheumatoid arthritis. See pages 82 and 89.

### 3. LEARN TO RELAX AND DEAL WITH STRESS
There is no doubt that rheumatoid arthritis is just one of many diseases that are made worse by stress and anxiety. Other forms of arthritis are also caused and exacerbated by stress. By learning how to combat stress – and how to relax thoroughly – you can improve your resistance and reduce your susceptibility to arthritis.

## Interferential Therapy

Unlike short wave diathermy and ultrasound, some experts claim that interferential therapy, another form of electrical treatment, does little to help speed up long-term recovery and is more likely to provide a short-term solution to pain. Like short wave diathermy and ultrasound this type of therapy is usually given two or three times a week for several weeks.

## Aids

Patients who are disabled by rheumatoid arthritis may be able to help themselves by using some or all of the aids or appliances described on pages 120–4.

## Case History

Michael had been an arthritis sufferer for eight years when he came to see me, complaining that the aspirin he was taking wasn't helping his joints at all. I was surprised by this news. Although he has quite severe rheumatoid arthritis, Michael has usually managed to keep his pain in check with nothing more complicated than ordinary soluble aspirin – a drug with which he feels comfortable. Michael has learned over the years how many tablets a day he can take without suffering from side effects such as dizziness, and he knows from bitter experience that some of the much more expensive replacements for aspirin can produce equally troublesome side effects.

When I examined Michael I could understand why he was complaining. His joints were more swollen and inflamed than usual and there were clear signs that his arthritis had flared up rather badly. We talked for quite a while and I could tell that Michael was upset about something.

Being well aware that stress and worry can make arthritis worse, I asked him if he had been under any unusual amount of stress recently. He coughed and started to tell me his story.

Michael ran a small, old-fashioned printing business with a partner. They had never made a lot of money, but they had always made enough to live on reasonably comfortably. I had never met Michael's partner, although I remembered hearing that his parents were extremely wealthy and owned a large bakery.

'My partner committed suicide four months ago,' said Michael suddenly. 'It was a terrible shock. I'd hardly got over that when I had another shock. Three weeks after my partner died, a man came to see me from a firm of solicitors. He was acting for a betting shop and he handed me a writ. I knew that Robert liked a bet but I had no idea just how far the addiction had gone and how much money he owed. The writ explained that Robert owed the betting shop a great deal of money and that because he and I were partners I was being held legally responsible for the debt. I was told that the printing business and Robert's home would have to be sold and warned that even then there probably would not be enough money to pay Robert's debts. The solicitor I went to see told me that I'll probably have to go into bankruptcy,' Michael told me.

It was pretty clear to me just why Michael's arthritis had flared up. The exceptional stress he was under had almost certainly had a dramatic effect on his immune system with the result that the rheumatoid arthritis had reached an unprecedented peak of pain and discomfort.

I prescribed a different anti-inflammatory drug for Michael, but I suspected that the stress Michael was under would continue to have a powerful influence on his body.

I asked Michael to come back and see me again in two weeks' time but he didn't appear. When a month had passed and I still hadn't seen Michael again, I called in at his home to see how he was. He wasn't there but Judy, his wife, was.

'Michael meant to ring you and let you know what happened,' she told me. 'He didn't come back to see you again because his arthritis settled down just as suddenly as it had flared up. I don't think it was the pills. In fact I don't even think Michael started them. But two days after he had been to see you our solicitor rang us to say that Robert's parents had been so upset when they had heard about what had happened that they had paid the bookmaker themselves. Robert's parents are going to keep Robert's share of the business but we don't have to sell it. You probably won't believe the difference it made to Michael,' she said. 'One day he could hardly walk, the next day he was back to normal.'

Stress is one of the most powerful causes of arthritis. There isn't always a quick solution, but many sufferers could help themselves if they learned how to reduce their exposure and increase their resistance to stress.

---

## WHAT CAN ALTERNATIVE THERAPISTS DO TO HELP COMBAT RHEUMATOID ARTHRITIS?

**Many types of alternative medicine can help you if you are a sufferer from Rheumatoid Arthritis. See pages 110–19 for more information.**

---

## HOW TO RELAX YOUR BODY

When you are anxious, nervous or under stress in any way your mind deliberately tenses up the muscles all over your body. There is a long-established, sensible reason for this. By tensing up muscles your mind is preparing your body for action; it assumes that the best way to deal with the threat you are facing will be physical action. Your mind is getting your body ready to fight or to run away.

But most modern stresses cannot be dealt with by a physical response. You cannot fight a traffic jam and running away from an electricity bill won't do you any good. Modern stresses persist for long periods – and so muscles remain tense for long periods too.

Tensed muscles commonly produce headaches, backache and stiff necks. Eight out of ten cases of backache are caused by stress and a staggering 98 per cent of headaches are produced in the same way.

Learning how to avoid unnecessary stresses,

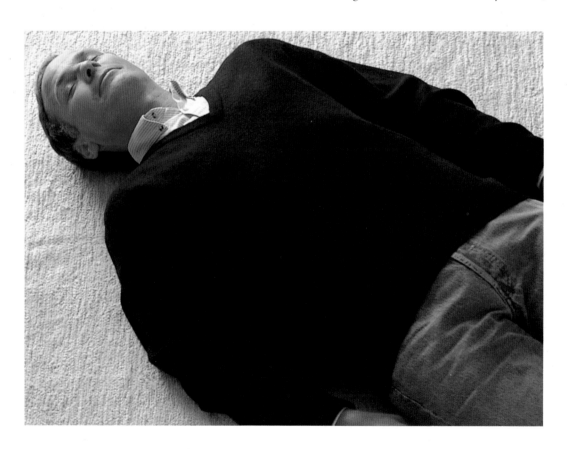

how to build up your resistance to stress and how to improve your ability to cope with stress will help you combat muscle tension.

But there is another, more direct, way to tackle muscle tension: deliberately relaxing your tensed muscles.

## RELAXATION TECHNIQUE

Make sure that you will not be disturbed for at least 20 minutes then lie down somewhere quiet and comfortable and use this simple-to-learn technique to help relieve muscle tension.

**1.** Take very deep, slow breaths. Stress will make you breathe much more quickly than usual so soothe your mind – and your body – by deliberately taking slower, deeper breaths.

**2.** Clench your left hand as tightly as you can, making a fist with your fingers. Do it well and you will see the knuckles go white. If you now let your fist unfold you will feel the muscles relax. When your hand was clenched the muscles were tensed; un-folded, the same muscles are relaxed. This is what you must do with the other muscle groups of your body.

**3.** Bend your left arm and try to make your left biceps muscle stand out as much as you can. Then relax it and let the muscles ease. When your arm is thoroughly relaxed let it lie loosely by your side.

**4.** Clench your right hand as tightly as you can, making a fist again with your fingers. When you let your fist unfold you will feel the muscles relax once more.

**5.** Now bend your right arm and make your right biceps muscle stand out as much as you can. Then relax it and let the muscles become relaxed. When your arm is thoroughly relaxed let it lie loosely by your side.

**6.** Tighten the muscles in your left foot. Curl your toes upwards, then downwards. When your foot feels as tense as you can make it deliberately relax the muscles.

**7.** Tense the muscles of your left calf. You should be able to feel the muscles in the back of your left leg become firm and hard as you tense them. Bend your foot up towards you to help tighten up the muscles. Then let the muscles relax.

**8.** Straighten your left leg and point your foot away from you. You will feel the muscles on the front of your left thigh tighten up – they should be firm right up to the top of your leg. Now relax those muscles and let your left leg lie loosely on the bed.

**9.** Tighten the muscles in your right foot. Curl your toes upwards towards your head and then downwards. When your foot feels as tense as you can make it you should deliberately relax the muscles.

**10.** Tense the muscles of your right calf. You should be able to feel the muscles in the back of your right leg become firm and hard as you tense them. Bend your foot up towards your head to help tighten the muscles. Then let the muscles relax.

**11.** Straighten your right leg and point your foot away from you. You will feel the muscles on the front of your right thigh tighten up – they should be firm right up to the top of your leg. Now relax those muscles and let your right leg lie loosely on the bed.

**12.** Lift yourself up by tightening your buttock muscles. You should be able to lift your body upwards by an inch or so. Then let your muscles fall loose again.

**13.** Tense and contract your abdominal muscles. Try to pull your abdominal wall in as far as possible. Then let go and allow your waist to reach its maximum circumference.

**14.** Tighten up the muscles of your chest. Take a big, deep breath in and strain to hold it for as long as possible. Then, very slowly, let your breath out.

**15.** Push your shoulders backwards as far as they will go, then bring them forwards and inwards. Finally, shrug them as high as you can. Keep your head perfectly still and try to touch your ears with your shoulders. It will probably be impossible but try anyway. Then let your shoulders relax and ease.

**16.** Next tighten up the muscles of your back. Try to make yourself as tall as you can. Then let the muscles relax.

**17.** The muscles of your neck are next. Lift your head forwards and pull at the muscles at the back of your neck. Turn your head first one way and then the other. Push your head backwards with as much force as you can. Then let the muscles of your neck relax. Move your head around and from side to side and make sure that your neck muscles are completely loose and easy.

**18.** Move your eyebrows upwards and then pull them down as far as they will go. Do this several times, making sure that you can feel the muscles tightening both when you move your eyebrows up and when you pull them down. Then let them relax.

**19.** Screw up your eyes as tightly as you are able to. Try to imagine that someone is trying to force your eyes open against your will. Keep them shut tightly. Then, keeping your eyelids closed, let them relax.

**20.** Move your lower jaw around. Grit your teeth. Wrinkle your nose. Smile as widely as you can, showing as many teeth as you can.

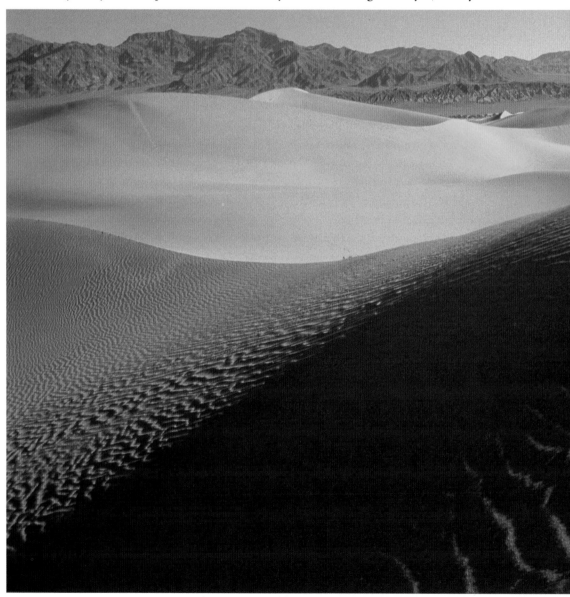

Push your tongue out as far as it will go. Push it firmly against the bottom of your mouth and then the top of your mouth before letting it lie easy and relaxed inside your mouth. Now let all your facial muscles go loose and relaxed.

## HOW TO RELAX YOUR MIND

We tend to think of our imaginations as light-hearted parts of our minds. That is a mistake that can prove deadly. The too often unrecognized truth is that the human imagination is powerful enough to kill. And the only person

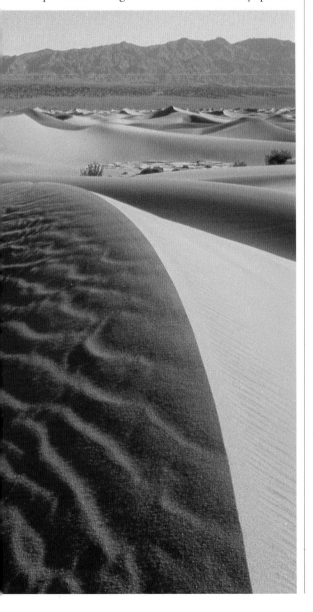

your imagination is likely to kill is you.

It is usually assumed that stress causes ill health because our bodies cannot cope with the strain of too much work, too much aggravation or too much excitement. But a good deal of the damage caused by stress is a consequence not of the real problems you may face but of the imaginary consequences your mind creates from those real problems.

For example, when you get up in the morning and find a telephone bill waiting for you, your immediate response will depend upon your ability to pay the bill. If you cannot pay the bill, the next response will be for your imagination to swing into action and to create a scenario detailing what might happen as a result of your inability to pay.

You may 'see' yourself being issued with a summons; being taken to court and publicly disgraced; being put in prison; losing your job; losing your home; losing your friends; being separated from your family and so on.

As you sit in your kitchen looking at the telephone bill none of these things are real. But once the telephone bill has triggered your imagination into action these imaginary consequences will have a very real effect on your body.

As you become increasingly worried and apprehensive so your blood pressure will rise, your muscles will become tense and acid will pour into your stomach to prepare your body for immediate action. In a very short time your imagination will have triggered an entirely inappropriate physical response. The result will probably be that within a few minutes you will end up with a headache or an attack of indigestion. It will not have been the telephone bill which will have done the damage, but your response to the arrival of the telephone bill; your headache won't be due to the piece of paper in your hand but to your imagination.

Have you ever watched a film in which there were long hot desert scenes? If you have then you've probably noticed that by the end of the film you felt quite thirsty. When that happened

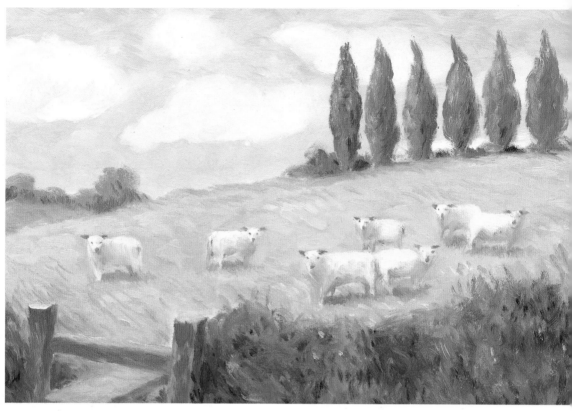

your body was responding to your imagination.

If you get an urgent message to ring someone close to you, your first reaction will probably be to worry. Your imagination will create a whole range of possible reasons for the telephone call. Maybe, you will think, there has been an accident. Perhaps someone has died. If you cannot get through on the telephone your mind will work overtime. Your imagination will create an endless series of possibilities. At the very least you will imagine a domestic crisis: a burst pipe or a fire in the kitchen. At the worst – well, at the worst your imagination will create a scenario far more horrendous than life could create. Your head will begin to ache, your muscles will tingle with tension and you will probably feel nauseated and shivery with apprehension.

When you eventually get through and speak to the caller and discover that they wanted to tell you that you had won a small amount of money in a lottery, your relief will be instant.

And yet all those seemingly terrible things that have been worrying you half to death only ever existed in the world of your imagination.

Your mind creates major stresses out of minor ones because your imagination creates a horrific scenario out of every small incident. It is hardly surprising that the vast majority of illnesses are caused or made worse by stress. It is hardly surprising that the pains and disablement of arthritis are often caused or made worse by the stress of twentieth-century life.

## RELAX YOUR MIND WITH A DAYDREAM

If you know how to do it you can harness the power of your imagination and use it to your advantage. In just the same way that your imagination can make you ill so it can also make you well again. All you have to do is to learn how – and that is no more difficult than learning how to swim or to ride a bicycle.

In order to take advantage of the healing powers of your imagination you must learn to fill your mind with peaceful and relaxing images.

Imagine it is a beautiful, warm, sunny day in

summer. The sky is blue and the only clouds are small, white and fluffy. You are driving along a twisting, turning country lane in a stylish, old, open-topped car. The lanes are deserted. All around you there are fields of golden corn dotted with scarlet poppies and hedgerows full of brightly coloured flowers.

You slow down, pull off the roadway on to a wide, grassy verge, turn off your engine and park and lock your car. Now you can hear the song birds singing in the hedgerow and the crickets chirping in the grass. The sunshine is warm but there is a gentle breeze to keep you cool.

You climb out of the car and walk across the gate towards a stile. On the other side of the stile there is a grassy meadow where a few young lambs are grazing. As though responding to some sixth sense the lambs look up for a moment and stare at you. Unworried and unhurried, they quickly settle down and carry on with their grazing.

Leisurely and easily you climb over the stile and into the meadow. You walk across the grass towards a small group of trees on the far side of the meadow. The lambs look up again, stare at you for a moment and then resume their constant chewing.

Suddenly, you are aware that there is a small river flowing nearby. You can hear the sound of water bubbling over a stone and gravel river bed. You walk along a narrow path that threads its way between a dozen huge oak trees and you slowly head down towards the source of the sound. It is cooler among the trees.

The river, which is wide and which flows slowly and peacefully, is the most beautiful stretch of water you have ever seen. You can see a kingfisher sitting on a branch on the other side of the river. A trout snaps lazily at a fly on the surface of the water. A moorhen, followed by a string of babies, paddles smoothly along the edge of the river, in and out of the reeds.

You sit down on an old tree stump, just in the shade, and watch the river flowing peacefully past you. A leaf drifts past. Then a twig. The family of moorhens turns noisily. The trout surfaces again. In a flash of blue the kingfisher swoops down from its branch and plucks a small fish out of the water.

You feel peaceful and relaxed and comfortable and happy and you do not have a care or a worry in the world.

If you allow yourself to drift wholeheartedly into this daydream then you should feel your muscles relaxing and your whole body becoming more comfortable. Your heartbeat will slow down and you will feel drowsy and content.

This sort of simple relaxation technique isn't difficult to learn, and it is an excellent way to combat stress and defeat anxiety.

## LEARN HOW TO DEAL WITH PAIN

Pain is one of the most common symptoms associated with rheumatoid arthritis. See Chapter 5.

## EXERCISE WHENEVER YOU CAN

You should not exercise when your joints are painful and inflamed, and you should avoid doing any exercise that hurts. But gentle, regular exercise that helps to keep your joints mobile, your muscles supple and strong and your body fit and healthy will dramatically improve your ability to overcome rheumatoid arthritis. See Chapter 7.

## HOW TO BUILD UP YOUR SELF-CONFIDENCE

Research done by psychologists have shown that arthritis sufferers tend to be rather timid and shy. They often come from unhappy homes and although they frequently build up a strong false front, arthritis sufferers are invariably obsessed with a sense of their own inferiority.

Psychologists have known for years that arthritis sufferers tend to treat themselves harshly; they are often dissatisfied with their own work; they push themselves far too hard and constantly search for a contentment and sense of personal satisfaction which escapes them.

Arthritis sufferers often feel inferior and helpless to change their own destiny. Here is a case history from my files which illustrates how one arthritis sufferer benefited by learning to build up her self confidence.

## CASE HISTORY

When Linda first came to see me she was in a terrible state. She had a bad skin rash on the backs of both of her hands and her asthma, from which she had suffered for most of her life, was almost out of control. She couldn't sleep and she was, she readily confessed, edgy and tearful all the time. Her long-standing arthritis was crippling her and she found it painful to walk.

'I just can't cope,' she told me, with tears forming in her eyes. 'I've got so much to do.'

I asked her to tell me exactly what she had to do and why she couldn't cope.

When she had finished explaining things to me I wasn't surprised that she was in a complete state. I don't think anyone could have coped with the workload she had acquired for herself. At the school where she worked as a teacher, Linda had taken on the responsibility of organizing the school play and of making all the arrangements for the summer fete. At the church she attended she had also been given the responsibility for organizing the fete. On top of all this she was trying to look after her aged and incontinent mother, her husband and her two teenage children. And to work full time as an art teacher.

'I feel so incompetent,' she sobbed. 'I know I ought to be able to do better but I just don't seem able to cope any more!"

'I'm not surprised!' I told her. 'You're trying to do far too much. Why did you allow yourself to be lumbered with so many jobs?'

Linda looked at me in some surprise and thought for a moment or two. 'I suppose its because I don't like to say "no",' she confessed.

And that was the key to Linda's problems. She didn't like to say 'no'.

'Why do you think you can't say "no"?' I asked her.

Linda thought for a long time before answering that question. 'I suppose it's because I don't like to let people down,' she replied. 'If I even think of saying "no" I always feel terribly guilty and end up saying "yes".'

I began to understand what forces were driving Linda to such a point of self destruction. The arthritis, the skin rash, the asthma, the sleeplessness and the tearfulness were all a result of the stress Linda was under, as a result of her apparently total inability to say 'no'.

As a child Linda's parents had been very ambitious for her. They had pushed her constantly and had never really been satisfied with her school work. Not once, Linda told me with tears streaming down her cheeks, had her parents ever praised her.

Linda had grown up desperately pushing herself harder and harder in a constant effort to please her unpleasable parents. When she had started work her total lack of self assurance and self confidence, and her constant search for appreciation and approval, meant that she took on all the jobs that no one else wanted to take on. She quickly acquired a reputation as an overwilling work horse.

And when she married the same thing happened again. Her husband, and then her children, learnt to be lazy and to let her do everything for them. She did all the shopping, all the cleaning, all the washing, all the ironing, all the cooking and all the washing up. She even did the gardening!

And driving her on all the time was her

### LEARN TO LET YOUR FEELINGS SHOW

**Arthritis sufferers often have difficulty in expressing their emotions. It seems likely that this inability to show emotion makes the development of arthritis more likely and makes symptoms worse when they do develop.**

burning need for approval from others. Everything she did was inspired by her deep rooted feeling of unworthiness.

I explained to Linda that the only long-term solution was for her to acquire more self esteem and self confidence.

'Only by building up your sense of self assurance and by learning that you have rights as well as responsibilities will you be able to escape from the treadmill you're on,' I told her.

Over the next few weeks I tried to show Linda how she could do just this.

First, I gave her a list of words to look at and I asked her to pick out any of the words which she thought applied to her.

Here is the list:

| | |
|---|---|
| • AGREEABLE | • SCRUPULOUS |
| • PUNCTILIOUS | • HONEST |
| • AMBITIOUS | • TRUTHFUL |
| • BRAVE | • RESPECTABLE |
| • CONSCIENTIOUS | • UNSELFISH |
| • CREATIVE | • OBEDIENT |
| • DECENT | • CAREFUL |
| • FAITHFUL | • BENEVOLENT |
| • LOYAL | • IMPECCABLE |
| • KIND | • HARD-WORKING |
| • INTELLIGENT | • THOUGHTFUL |
| • POLITE | • WISE • |

'Oh, I don't think any of those apply to me,' said Linda.

'Of course they do!" I insisted. 'You're unselfish, aren't you! And you're respectable'

'Yes, I suppose so.' She paused and nodded. 'I suppose I am,' she agreed.

'And you will agree you are truthful and polite and benevolent?'

Linda agreed, after hesitating, that these words did accurately describe her.

'And you're attentive and agreeable and conscientious and careful?'

Again Linda thought carefully. And then, when she had thought about it, again she nodded. Gradually, I managed to convince her

that she did have many excellent qualities. Indeed, by the time we had finished going through the list, Linda had to agree that most of the words applied to her.

'But none of that makes me a good person,' said Linda. 'I'm always getting things wrong. I always seem to be making mistakes. And I just don't seem to be able to cope.'

'What sort of things do you tend to get wrong? In what way don't you think you can cope?' I asked.

'Well, I bought the wrong sort of tea for my mother the other day and she didn't like it one bit. And my daughter went mad at me because I didn't have her jeans ironed in time for her to go out on Saturday.' She stopped and looked down at her lap. 'I always seem to have to be apologizing,' she said sadly. She shrugged. 'It happens all the time.'

'How old is your daughter?' I asked her.

'Fifteen.'

'Is she handicapped?'

Linda looked up at me. 'No.'

'Why didn't she iron her jeans herself?'

Linda looked puzzled at this; she had clearly never even thought of asking her daughter to help with the ironing.

'Why does it always have to be you who does everything?" I asked her. 'You are making yourself ill by trying so hard to do things to please other people.'

I explained to Linda that no one can do everything and that there is, in any case, no shame in making mistakes or getting things wrong occasionally.

'You need to be more selfish,' I told her. 'How much time in the week do you have to do things that you want to do?'

Linda looked at me as if I were mad. 'What do you mean?'

'When did you last do something that was just for you'.

Linda frowned. She couldn't think of anything.

'You let people push you around because you

are constantly searching for approval, and because you've got absolutely no self respect or self assurance', I explained. 'And because you are trying to do the impossible and please everyone all of the time your health is beginning to suffer.' I explained to her that disorders such as arthritis, asthma and eczema often attack individuals who are self effacing and who allow themselves to be pushed around by others.

'You must learn not to worry too much about occasional mistakes,' I told her. 'And there is absolutely nothing at all wrong or shaming about having to say "I was wrong" or "I made a mistake" occasionally. The only people who never have to say they were wrong are the people who never do anything, who never try anything and who never take any risks.'

Slowly, Linda began to realize that she was not a bad person but that she was a weak person, and that she was being pushed around.

Gradually, I managed to get Linda to realize that she had many wonderful qualities; that she was kind and thoughtful and generous. I managed to persuade her to begin to think about herself a little more often; to take charge of at least part of her own life and to say "no" occasionally to people.

Eventually, Linda came into the surgery one Saturday with a broad smile on her face.

'What happened?' I asked her.

'My daughter brought some friends home today," said Linda. 'And when she found that I hadn't had time to do the washing up after breakfast so she couldn't make her friends a cup of coffee she came storming in to complain.'

'What did you do?' I asked her.

'I told her that I was busy and that if she wanted clean cups she could wash some up herself," said Linda, looking both slightly pleased with herself and slightly embarrassed by her own cheek. I couldn't help noticing that her skin rash had cleared up.

'What did she do?'

'She washed up some cups!' said Linda, unable to contain her delight.

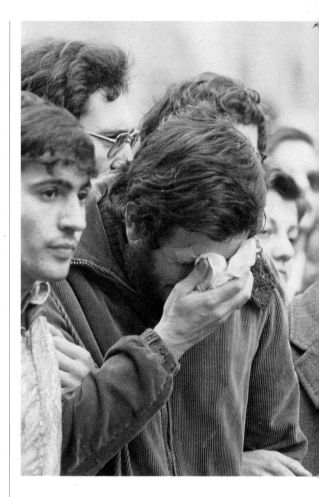

*Crying is a healthy way to respond to sadness.*

Linda will probably never be completely free of her ingrained desire to please other people. But she has, at least, made a start.

And when she left the surgery that day and I asked her how her arthritis was she turned and looked at me as though she didn't know what I was talking about.

'What arthritis?' she asked.

## CRYING IS GOOD FOR YOU

I firmly believe that one of the main reasons why Italian men suffer less from heart disease than do British men (despite the fact that many of them eat the wrong foods, are overweight, drink too much and smoke too much) is that the former aren't afraid to cry. British boys are taught that it is unmanly to cry. At school and at home they learn that crying is a girlish, wimpy thing to do. They are taught that they must respond to sadness, sorrow and despair with a stiff upper lip; they are taught to 'bottle up' their natural emotions and to pretend that everything is all right. The boy or man who does cry will suffer twice: first, he will suffer the original pain and then he will suffer from a sense of guilt and shame for having given way to tears.

Countless male leaders in Britain, America and Australia have lost credibility and respect through having cried in public. And yet crying is an important and effective way of dealing with stress; it is one of the body's most important ways of dealing with problems and pressures and it is, above all, an absolutely natural way of dealing with sadness.

When a baby cries it is making it clear to its parents that it desperately wants love and attention. When a child falls over in the garden and runs in crying to its mother it is making it clear that it wants reassurance and comfort. A mother who sees her child crying will pick it up, cuddle it, give it affection and show that she cares. The tears will attract sympathy and support when they are most needed.

The man who refuses to cry because he believes that it is a sign of weakness is putting himself at risk. By hiding his emotions he will turn a short-term sadness into a long-term frustration and exchange a temporary despair for a permanent depression.

Men who never cry are far more likely to suffer from stress-related disorders such as heart disease, high blood pressure, stomach ulcers and arthritis than are men who allow the tears to flow when they feel sad. It is now well known that people who suffer from arthritis are quite likely to have difficulty in expressing their emotions.

The man who hides his tears and turns his sadness inwards is storing up trouble for the future; by crying, and allowing his sadness to show, he would attract the love and the sympathy that can heal sadness; by refusing to cry he is making himself ever more vulnerable to unhappi-ness and ensuring that he will become yet another victim of stress.

In recent years scientists have managed to confirm that crying is good for us. We know now that as well as attracting love and sympathy, crying helps by getting rid of potentially dangerous chemical waste products which would otherwise build up in the body and lead to the development of long-term depression.

When you cry because you are sad your tears are different to the tears you shed when you cry because you have something in your eye. Scientists have discovered that the tears which are triggered by sadness have a different physical content to the tears which are inspired by specks of dust or gusts of wind.

Everyone should learn to cry when they feel sad; crying is nothing to be ashamed of – it is, rather, a natural and healthy response which invariably leads to a sense of contentment and a calmness which would otherwise be unattainable.

## DEAL POSITIVELY WITH ANGER

People who suffer from arthritis often have difficulty in showing their anger. They feel bad about letting other people know how they feel and so they hide their angry feelings deep inside their souls. In the end, of course, that anger will show itself in some way or other – often by doing permanent damage to the joints.

Arthritis sufferers frequently feel that if they give expression to their anger they will be exhibiting some weakness.

The fact of the matter, of course, is altogether different.

The truth is that we all feel angry occasionally. Even the most placid and peaceful person sometimes feels cross about some injustice or is driven to anger by some series of frustrations.

And the healthiest solution is often to show that anger – to let it out.

If you hold your anger inside you, and refuse to let it out, then in the end you will almost undoubtedly damage yourself in some way.

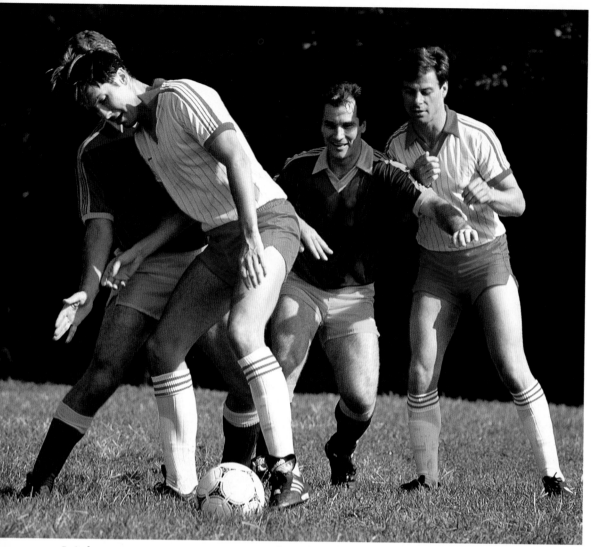

*It is better to express your anger in some harmless physical way than to bottle it up*

Of course, I do not recommend letting your anger out in an unsociable or illegal fashion – that would merely lead to more frustrations and more injustices and more sadness and more anger! But there are lots of quite practical ways in which it is possible to get rid of accumulated anger in a healthy and useful way.

For example, you may be able to get rid of your anger by performing some exhausting physical task. Maybe you have a garden you can dig (though if you do, then please be careful not to do too much too quickly – every year thousands of men and women injure their joints and give themselves backache by being too enthusiastic in the garden) or maybe you can give the house a good spring clean.

Many people get rid of their anger through exercise. Maybe you could go to the gym and work out, or attend an aerobics class, or go swimming or for a run, or play a game of squash, tennis or football.

Whatever you choose to do you should, of course, remember that you must not allow your anger to make you forget all the safety precautions you have learnt. If you allow your anger to push you too hard then you will find it all too easy to damage a joint or to injure yourself – or someone else – in some way.

## LEARN TO LAUGH

You may find it difficult to believe but there is now plenty of evidence to show that laughter can help overcome arthritis. For example, consider the case of Peter.

Peter had been a patient of mine for years and he suffered from terrible arthritis which made it difficult for him to move about. His spine, his arms and his legs were all affected to some degree or another. Over the years Peter had tried many different treatments for his arthritis but, sadly, none of the treatments he had tried had worked very well.

Even before he had contracted arthritis, Peter had been a rather unhappy man. He had never been a lighthearted person who laughed readily. He simply didn't seem to have a particularly well-developed sense of humour.

I talked to him about this one day and suggested that he should consciously try to develop his sense of humour by watching amusing films and reading funny books. He decided to take up my suggestion and went out and rented a Marx Brothers video. It was, for him, a revelation.

Peter had never, ever sat down and made time to watch something funny. He had never allowed himself to laugh before. But the Marx Brothers film converted him. The first sight of Harpo Marx, the first unwilling giggle, changed his life. He then went on to discover comedians he had never heard of before. For Peter, laughter really was the best medicine.

Within weeks his arthritis was less troublesome. It didn't go away completely; some days it still troubles him. But it is much, much better than it has been for years.

## TRY OLIVE OIL!

When doctors treated patients suffering from rheumatoid arthritis with olive oil they found that they needed fewer drugs to control their pain and stiffness. The doctors therefore concluded that olive oil may have a direct anti-inflammatory effect on arthritic joints.

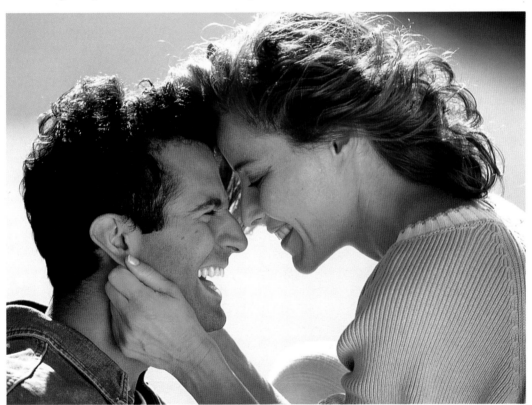

*It's an old adage, but there is a strong element of truth in it – laughter is the best medicine.*

# CHAPTER THREE

# Osteoarthritis

*Osteoarthritis usually first affects people in their fifties or sixties. It seems to appear in women slightly more often than in men and usually affects the joints of the spine, the knees, hips, hands and feet.*

## CAUSES AND SYMPTOMS

At the beginning of the disease there is usually only one joint affected but as time goes by osteoarthritis can spread to many parts of the body. Unlike rheumatoid arthritis (to which it bears remarkably few similarities other than that both are joint diseases), osteoarthritis does not involve damage to other parts of the body. It is a much simpler disease to understand than rheumatoid arthritis.

The main symptoms are stiffness and aching which develop as the cartilage between the bones gradually gets thinner and thinner. Eventually the bones end up rubbing on one another.

Osteoarthritis can be caused by excess wear and tear (in which case it is practically indistinguishable from the problems often caused by old age) but it can be inherited and may affect younger adults.

## WHAT ARE THE CAUSES OF OSTEOARTHRITIS?

We reach our physical peak in our late teens and early twenties and from then on it is, I'm afraid, all downhill! Our vision becomes less acute, our hearing more indistinct and our brains lose nerve cells at a frightening rate. After the age of 40 our bones become weaker and more likely to fracture, our muscles lose some of their strength and our joints stiffen up and start to creak a little. Most of these changes are gradual and painless and go unnoticed until we suddenly try to do something that we used to be able to do with ease and find that our bodies let us down.

It is the changes inside our joints which so often lead to the development of osteoarthritis.

As explained on pages 9–14, a normal healthy joint is perfectly designed for the job it has to do. Those joints which have a synovium and are filled with synovial fluid are particularly impressive from an engineering point of view: they are strong and they have a self-lubricating system which cannot be matched by modern designers with their computers and sophisticated oils. Each one of the synovial joints in a normal, healthy body is more slippery and efficient than any man-made joint could ever hope to be.

## SYNOVIAL JOINTS HAVE THREE SPECIAL ATTRIBUTES

The synovial fluid inside the joint is made of a special substance which loses water and becomes thicker when the pressure on the joint is greater. This means that the lubricant automatically becomes more efficient and more protective when the need for lubrication is at its greatest.

The two cartilaginous surfaces of a synovial joint are extraordinarily slippery and would move smoothly together even without a lubricant. Cartilage grows gradually throughout childhood and in adulthood it can, to a small extent, heal itself if it is injured or replace itself if it wears away.

Although the cartilaginous surfaces look smooth they are full of tiny indentations, rather like a golf ball. The result is that synovial fluid is

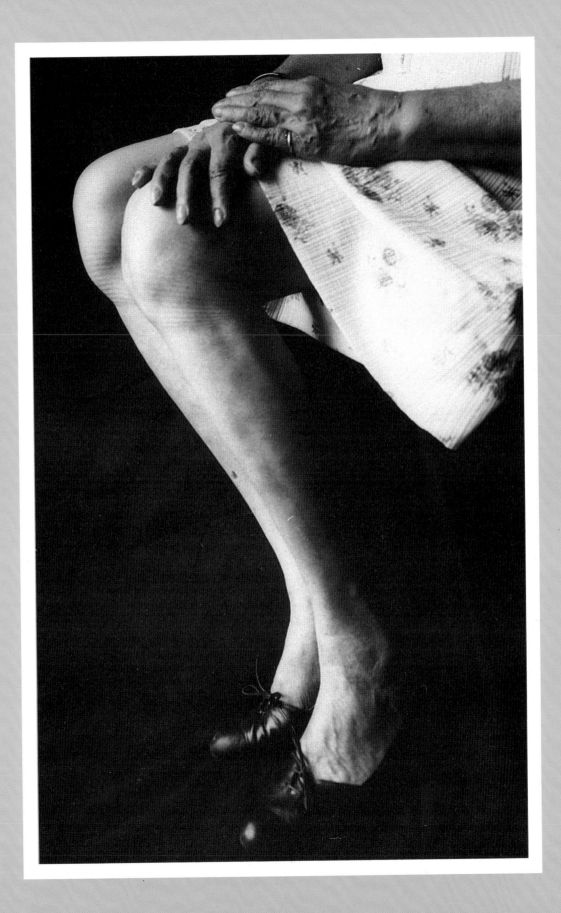

trapped between the two surfaces, thereby reducing the amount of friction still further.

To get an idea of the amount of work each of your joints has to do, just stop and think of the number of times that you move your arms and legs in an ordinary day. Getting up, sitting down, picking things up and walking about all put a pressure on your joints.

Obviously, all this action means that our joints begin to wear out faster than they can repair themselves, and that is often what happens as we get older. Our cartilages wear down too quickly and the production of lubricating fluid becomes a little sluggish.

But although osteoarthritis may be partly a consequence of ageing that is not by any means the whole story.

For a start, most of us are so accustomed to the fact that our joints are strong, resilient and hard-wearing that we do very little to look after them or to help protect them from unnecessary wear and tear.

The worst thing that most of us do to damage our joints is to allow ourselves to become overweight. If you are 14 lb (6.3 kg) overweight then your joints will be constantly carrying an unnecessary load. Try picking up 14 lb (6.3 kg) of sugar or flour and walking around with it for five minutes or so. That is what your joints have to put up with for every minute of your waking day. The heavier you are – and the more excess weight you are carrying – the greater the strain on your joints will be. If you are overweight then the chances are high that it will be the joints in your hips, knees and ankles – your weight-bearing joints – which suffer from osteoarthritis first.

We make things even worse by taking exercise that puts a tremendous strain on our bodies, by battering our bones and cartilages and by putting totally unreasonable demands on the resilience of our joints.

*"After the age of 40 our bones become weaker and more likely to fracture, and our muscles lose some of their strength."*

When we are young our bones are capable of absorbing an enormous amount of stress, but as we age they become less elastic and less capable of taking any sort of punishment. The result is that your joints have to take increasing amounts of the shock when you walk, run, jump, dance or leap about. Your joints are at their best when you are about 20 years old. Every year after that means a year's additional decay. By the time you are 30 your joints may be noticeably stiffer and more vulnerable. After the age of 40, weight-bearing joints in particular are likely to start creaking and causing trouble.

Jogging, running, tennis, squash, football and aerobics all put a tremendous strain on your joints (particularly if you are not wearing shock-absorbing foot-wear). And, of course, if you are overweight then the strain will be increased.

Although osteoarthritis is usually a consequence of old age or over-use it is not always a result of natural wear and tear. Sometimes osteoarthritis may develop in younger people who are not overweight and who have done relatively little exercise. When this happens it may be because salts have been deposited in the cartilages, because inflammation or infection has damaged the joint or because the two parts of a joint do not fit together properly as a result of some congenital abnormality (the hip joint being the one that is most commonly affected by congenital problems).

## WHO GETS OSTEOARTHRITIS?

Anyone can get osteoarthritis – at any age – but it doesn't usually start before the age of 30 or 40 years old and it is most common after the age of 50. It affects women more than men and, although it is so common that it is difficult to be certain about this, it does seem to affect some families more than others. People who are over-weight are prone to osteoarthritis and if you have ever had an injury in a joint you will be more likely to get osteoarthritis in that joint.

## How Common Is Osteoarthritis?

It is difficult to say how many people get osteoarthritis because most sufferers manage without seeking medical help. However, millions are severely disabled by osteoarthritis and it is probably the commonest cause of disability in the Western world.

## How Quickly Does Osteoarthritis Develop?

It is rare for osteoarthritis to develop quickly; it usually starts slowly and builds up gradually over a period of years. Sometimes it develops so slowly that a sufferer may become quite crippled without ever really noticing or complaining of any severe pain or disablement. It is, however, possible for an injury (even a relatively minor one) to exacerbate osteoarthritis in a joint.

## Which Joints Does Osteoarthritis Affect?

Osteoarthritis normally only affects joints below the waist. The hips, knees, ankles, hands and feet are the joints most commonly affected. Sometimes some of the joints in the back may be affected. Occasionally, only one joint will be affected by osteoarthritis but it is more common for two or three joints to be involved.

### The Hips

The hip is a ball and socket joint which has a wide range of movement (only the shoulder joint has a wider range). Because it is an important weight-bearing joint it is the most common joint in the body to be affected by osteoarthritis. People who are overweight are particularly likely to be affected. When osteoarthritis develops in the hip it causes increasing stiffness and even the slightest movement may be painful. Walking can

be very difficult and even movements in bed can cause excruciating pain. When a hip is affected by osteoarthritis it gradually changes in shape and the end result can be that the leg on that side may effectively become noticeably shorter than the other leg – making walking particularly difficult and putting an additional strain on the rest of the body. Because people who have damaged hips may be unable to move about enough to look after themselves properly osteoarthritis of the hip is by far the commonest single cause of disablement today.

### The Knees

Osteoarthritis in the knees can cause a wide range of deformities. It can make the knees look knobbly and make the sufferer appear bow legged or knock-kneed. Patients with osteoarthritis of the knees often have difficulty in walking up and down stairs. It is possible to hear creaking and grating noises whenever osteoarthritic knee joints are moved.

### The Ankles

Although they have to carry the weight of the whole body the ankles are less likely than the hips or knees to develop osteoarthritis – possibly because the normal range of movement in the ankle joint is less than that of the hips or knees and the amount of wear and tear is, therefore, considerably less. The ankle joint is only responsible for up and down movements of the foot – other movements (such as rotating and tilting) are produced by joints within the foot.

### The Feet

The most common joint in the foot to be affected by osteoarthritis is the joint at the base of the big toe. Problems are usually caused by long-term pressure produced by shoes that don't fit properly. Women – who are more likely to wear shoes that are designed to look fashionable rather than to provide the feet with any protection or support – are far more likely to suffer from this type of osteoarthritis than men are.

### THE SHOULDERS

The shoulders are only rarely affected by osteoarthritis, and usually only after injury.

### THE ELBOWS

Like the shoulders, the elbows are only rarely affected by osteoarthritis – and, again, usually only after injury. The rarity of osteoarthritis in the shoulders and the elbows shows quite clearly just how important excess weight can be in the development of osteoarthritis of the knees and hips (which are joints of similar design and a similar range of movements).

### THE HANDS

In the hands, osteoarthritis most commonly affects the joint at the base of the thumb and those at the ends of the fingers. Small, hard nodules often form at the backs of affected joints in the hand and although these are usually painless they can add to the stiffness of the joints.

## WHAT ARE THE SYMPTOMS OF OSTEOARTHRITIS?

Pain is by far the most important symptom of osteoarthritis and can vary from a dull and persistent but often bearable ache to a sharp, gnawing pain. Usually worse after joints have been used a lot (that invariably means at the end of the day), the pain of osteoarthritis is produced when pain endings in the bones and ligaments are stimulated. The dull, deep and generalized ache in and around the affected joints is caused by changes in the pressure within the bones – which is itself a result of the failure of the joint to function properly. The sharper, more acute pain of osteoarthritis is usually produced when a ligament catches on or is stretched by a piece of irregular bone in the joint. In addition to these 'internal' pains there may sometimes be a feeling of tenderness over an affected joint.

The second significant symptom of osteoarthritis is stiffness, which is usually worst in the mornings or after any period of rest or inactivity. Most sufferers of osteoarthritis find that their joints are worse if they spend a long time in the same position. Regular, gentle movements of a joint help to keep stiffness at bay, although when a joint is affected by osteoarthritis its range of movement is usually less than the range of movement in a perfectly healthy joint.

Finally, there may be some swelling of osteoarthritic joints. In particular, nodules may appear around the finger joints and the knee joints may swell as fluid accumulates.

## OSTEOARTHRITIS IS FOR LIFE

Osteoarthritis does not usually come and go and nor does it have 'active' and 'inactive' phases in the way that rheumatoid arthritis does. Usually, once a joint develops osteoarthritis it remains osteoarthritic for life.

## JOINT DAMAGE MAY RESULT IN DISABLEMENT

Osteoarthritis is a major cause of disablement. Since it is the knees and hips which are most commonly affected sufferers often have difficulty in walking, bending and stretching. They may also have difficulty in getting into and out of soft, 'comfortable' chairs.

## OSTEOARTHRITIS CAN CAUSE INACTIVITY AND DEPRESSION

Because osteoarthritis causes disablement and makes mentally alert individuals immobile it commonly also causes depression.

## WHAT TESTS CAN BE DONE FOR OSTEOARTHRITIS?

X-ray pictures of suspected joints will show how much damage has been done, what changes there have been to the bones and whether there is any narrowing of the joint space between the bones. Blood tests are of limited value but doctors sometimes take a sample of fluid from a joint to check for any signs of inflammation and to see if there are any crystals present in the joint (see gout on page 64).

## CAN OSTEOARTHRITIS BE TREATED ?

Osteoarthritis cannot be 'cured' by any miracle pills (although surgeons can replace a damaged joint with a 'new' one) but there are ways in which the symptoms can be controlled and the development of the disease can be minimized.

## WHAT CAN DOCTORS DO TO HELP COMBAT OSTEOARTHRITIS?

## DRUGS

Drugs will not cure osteoarthritis nor will they affect the progress of the disease, but they can relieve pain and help keep joints mobile and so avoid further stiffening. Pain-killers such as aspirin and paracetamol are most commonly prescribed. By relieving pain and combating inflammation they help to reduce the amount of stiffness patients have to deal with.

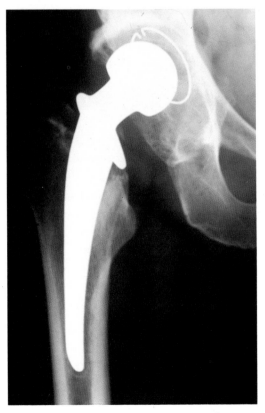

*A hip replacement can give an osteoarthritis patient a new life free of disability.*

Many doctors also prescribe other drugs in the non-steroidal anti-inflammatory group. Steroids are unlikely to be useful in the treatment of osteoarthritis since the symptoms are mainly caused by wear and tear within the joint rather than by inflammation.

## SUPPOSITORIES

See entry in Chapter Two on page 27.

## INJECTIONS

Injections can be performed to remove excess fluid and, if there is any inflammation in the joint, a steroid injection may be useful.

## SURGERY

Since the 1960s surgeons around the world have been replacing osteoarthritic hip joints with artificial joints and today hip replacement operations are commonplace and immensely successful. Indeed, hip replacement surgery has been so successful that many surgeons are now replacing other joints – particularly knees and joints in the hands.

The operation to remove and replace an osteoarthritic hip joint is relatively safe and straightforward to perform (it has been done on patients in their nineties). A metal and plastic replacement is glued into the patient's own bones. The success rate is high, with most patients standing up a day or two after the operation and walking within two or three weeks. Advances are constantly being made in the design of joint replacements and, in particular, in the type of materials used to provide an effective long-life replacement. It is, as you can imagine, difficult to mimic the efficiency of the human joint but artificial joints are now being made that can last for 15 years of relatively active movement.

Joint replacement is not the only type of surgery which is offered to patients with osteoarthritis. Sometimes it is possible to cut through the bone near to an osteoarthritic joint and to take pressure off the joint by realigning the bone. This type of operation is called an osteotomy and in addition to removing pain and pressure from the area it can also stimulate the body to heal itself.

## PHYSIOTHERAPY

A physiotherapist can help to reduce pain and stiffness and to keep joints mobile. See page 29.

## AIDS

If you are disabled in any way by osteoarthritis you will be able to retain your independence by using some of the many available aids and appliances. See pages 120–4 for more details.

## HOW CAN ALTERNATIVE THERAPISTS HELP COMBAT OSTEOARTHRITIS?

Because osteoarthritis is a disease that is usually caused by wear and tear within the joint there is little that alternative or complementary therapists can do to provide permanent relief of the symptoms. However, some alternative therapies are capable of helping to relieve pain, and many patients have found that acupuncture in particular is extremely good for this. See page 112 for more details on acupuncture.

## WHAT CAN YOU DO TO HELP COMBAT OSTEOARTHRITIS?

### LOSE EXCESS WEIGHT

If you stop to think about it then it makes perfect sense that if you have arthritis of any kind you should try to lose any excess weight. Try walking around the house carrying a 2 lb (1 kg) bag of sugar and multiply that by the amount you are overweight. If you are 14 lb (6.3 kg) overweight you are effectively carrying around with you seven bags of sugar – all the time!

Osteoarthritis, which commonly affects large, weight-bearing joints such as the hips and knees, is likely to be made worse if you are overweight.

Sadly, most of the people who try to lose

weight fail. Even if they lose weight successfully in the short term most will put all their weight back on again within a few months.

They fail because instead of changing their bad eating habits they try to lose weight by going on unnatural diets. Then, when they go back to their former eating habits, they simply put all the weight back on again.

If you are going to lose weight permanently you really have to make sure that you change your eating habits permanently.

Here are two pieces of valuable advice which should help you lose your excess, unwanted weight – and keep it off!

### SET YOURSELF A MANAGEABLE TARGET

Most slimmers start off by setting themselves impossible targets. They decide how much they need to lose and then aim to lose all of that excess weight – which they may have accumulated over a period of years – in just a few weeks. I once organized a survey of slimmers and discovered to my absolute horror that around nine out of every ten were aiming at a target weight that was far too low for them. Worse still, all of them were hoping to lose their weight at a completely unrealistic rate.

The problem with setting yourself an impossible target is that you will almost certainly fail. And then, when you fail, you will be depressed; you will think of yourself as a slimming failure and you will probably abandon your plans to lose weight. Failure breeds failure and once a would-be slimmer has failed she (or he) will probably just give up, abandon all hope and put up with her (or his) excess weight.

So, the first thing you should do is to set yourself a realistic target.

If you look at the height weight tables I have prepared you will be able to find the ideal weight band for your height. I have deliberately created tables which are fairly broad because people are different. Some people do have slightly heavier bones than others and some have a naturally

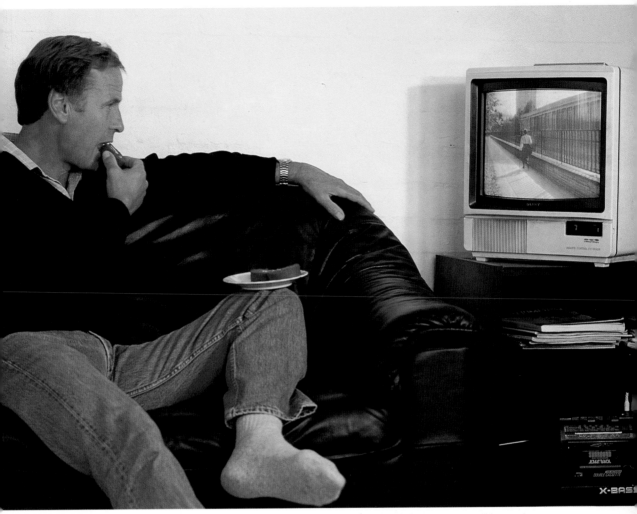

*If you eat while watching television you won't be aware of your appetite control centre.*

'heavier' body build. You should aim to be somewhere within (or close to) the ideal weight band for your height but don't try to be the same weight at 40 as you were when you were 20 and don't aim at model-like slenderness if you are in your fifties and a grandmother of seven. There is no point at all in setting yourself an unrealistic target – all you are likely to do is to make yourself feel a failure.

Once you have decided roughly how much you should weigh you can, of course, simply subtract that from your current weight to find out how much you need to lose. Then, since you should aim at losing around 2lb (1 kg) a week, divide the total amount of weight you need to

lose by two to find the number of weeks that your weight loss programme should last.

I know that this may sound a slow way of losing weight but even if you only lose 2 lb (1 kg) a week you will be able to lose a massive 26 lb (11.7 kg) in three months and 52 lb (23.4 kg) in six months.

Once you've worked out your long-term target give yourself some short-term aims. Decide, for example, that you are going to try to lose 8 lb (3.6 kg) in the next month. And then weigh yourself just once a week to check on your progress. (Don't weigh yourself too often – your weight will fluctuate naturally from day to day and if you weigh yourself several times a day as

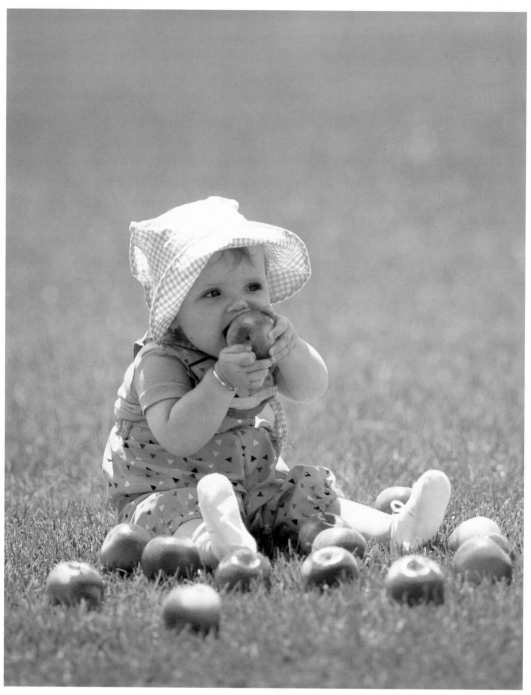

*Experiments have shown that children, when offered a choice of foods, will choose a healthy diet.*

some people do, then you will probably depress yourself when you realize that your weight sometimes goes up a little when you think it ought to be going down).

The big advantage of this simple approach is that every time you hit a small and realistic slimming target you will think of yourself as a success. Every time you lose a bit more of your unwanted weight you will feel like a winner. And once you feel like a successful slimmer your confidence will be boosted and you will tackle your next target with renewed enthusiasm.

## ONLY EAT
## WHEN YOU ARE HUNGRY

In October 1928 Dr Clara M. Davis of Chicago published the results of one of the most remarkable human experiments ever conducted. The results of the experiment were published in the *American Journal of Diseases.*

Dr Davis had three aims when she started her experiment. She wanted to know whether young, newly weaned infants could:

**a) select foods which would help them to stay healthy**

**b) choose their own food and eat enough to stay alive**

**c) select a good, well-balanced diet without any outside help.**

Dr Davis found that without any prompting the infants she had chosen for her experiment automatically chose good, varied diets when they were allowed to decide for themselves what they wanted to eat. Their growth rates, development, vigour and appearance were all just as good as those of babies who had been eating diets carefully organized by expert nutritionists and dieticians. Amazingly, the young children in Dr Davis's experiment, who were merely following their natural eating instincts, ate the right types of food in just the right amounts – and, therefore, they stayed healthy.

Dr Davis's experiment was, I believe, one of the most remarkable research projects ever described and it led the way to the discovery of the appetite control centre – an extremely impressive and powerful automatic device which is hidden deep inside every human brain. The power of the appetite control centre is quite remarkable; it can make sure that you never become short of essential vitamins and minerals and it can make sure that you never weigh too much or too little.

All you have to do to take advantage of your appetite control centre is to learn to listen to it!

Just five years after her original experiment Dr Davis published the results of some more research. Having studied a total of 15 young children for between six months and four and a half years, she came to the conclusion that although none of the children in the experiment had been told what to eat they all remained healthy. To the experts their eating habits seemed unplanned, even chaotic, but none of the children suffered from anything that could be related to food. There were no stomach aches and no constipation and none of the children in this experiment became fat.

The experiment proved again that when children are allowed to select what they eat for themselves they choose a very sensible diet.

During the Second World War a large and slightly more sophisticated experiment was conducted by a group of army doctors. The results demonstrated the same principle: that when soldiers are allowed access to unlimited supplies of food they eat precisely what their bodies need according to their environment! When they were allowed to eat what they liked the soldiers automatically chose – without any professional guidance – a mixture of fat, protein and carbohydrate that was exactly right for their nutritional needs.

*"The secret of permanent slimming success is to eat when you are hungry – and to stop when you are no longer hungry."*

## LISTEN TO YOUR BODY

I have mentioned all these experiments because you can learn a lot from them.

The conclusion must be that if you listen to your body – and you learn to eat when your body tells you to and to stop eating when it tells you to stop – then you will not go far wrong. If, in addition, you can make sure that you eat the foods your body tells you to eat, you will not only stay slim but you will also stay healthy.

I have explained the virtues and values of this

simple system to numerous slimmers and everyone who has had even the smallest amount of determination needed to try it out has succeeded – and has lost weight permanently. As far as I know there has never been a single failure.

This system is beautifully simple, it is foolproof, it doesn't cost any money, there are no side-effects and it is permanent. It is hardly surprising if the only problem with it is that some people think it sounds too good to be true.

'Why,' ask the sceptics, 'am I fat if my brain already contains an appetite control centre that is supposed to keep me slim?'

There is a simple answer to that apparently difficult question.

The truth is that most of us have lost the art of listening to our own bodies. We have, sadly, acquired many bad eating habits and we allow these to overrule our internal appetite control centre. We eat for all sorts of 'bad' reasons.

We eat not because we are hungry but because we are bored (and food provides us with excitement); because we are depressed (and eating cheers us up) and because we are guilty (and food helps us to forget our guilt). We eat at fixed meal times (whether we are hungry or not) because we have been taught to eat at fixed meal times. We finish up all the food on our plates (whether or not we need it) because when we were small we were told about the starving millions – and reminded that they would be grateful for the food we were leaving. We eat more than we need because when we were bottle fed our mothers taught us to empty the bottle – rather than to listen to our own appetite control centres telling us that we were full.

And so it goes on.

Over the years we acquire many bad eating habits. We ignore our appetite control centres. And so we end up getting fat.

The secret of permanent slimming success is to eat when you are hungry – and to stop eating when you are no longer hungry.

Because I realize that slimming isn't easy – even when you know the secret of slimming success – I have prepared a special slimming tape script to help you.

## THE SLIMMING TAPE

I suggest that you record your own tape on a cassette recorder and then play back the tape you have made every morning and evening so that you give your determination and your willpower a daily boost. After a week you may find that listening to the tape just once a day is enough.

When you record the tape I suggest that you speak as slowly and as clearly as you can. If you know someone who has a voice you like listening to you might like to try getting them to record the tape for you.

When you listen to the tape try to find somewhere quiet where you won't be disturbed. Shut the door and maybe even take the telephone off the hook. You may find that the tape works better if you listen to it on a personal stereo with just a pair of headphones rather than a loudspeaker system.

### THE SCRIPT FOR YOUR PERSONAL SLIMMING TAPE

Close your eyes and take big, slow, deep breaths. To make sure that you breathe in slowly try counting up to four while you are breathing in.

Then, hold your breath and count up to two.

And then breathe out slowly, counting up to four as you breathe out.

When your lungs are empty stay like that while you count up to two and then repeat the process again. Take another deep breath, counting up to four while you are breathing in; hold your breath and count up to two; breathe out slowly, counting up to four as you breathe out; and when your lungs are empty count up to two.

By breathing in and out slowly and deeply you should be able to relax your body.

Next, when you feel that your body is relaxed, you must try to relax your mind.

Try to imagine that you are lying on a sunny beach on a glorious midsummer's day.

To the left and to the right there is endless

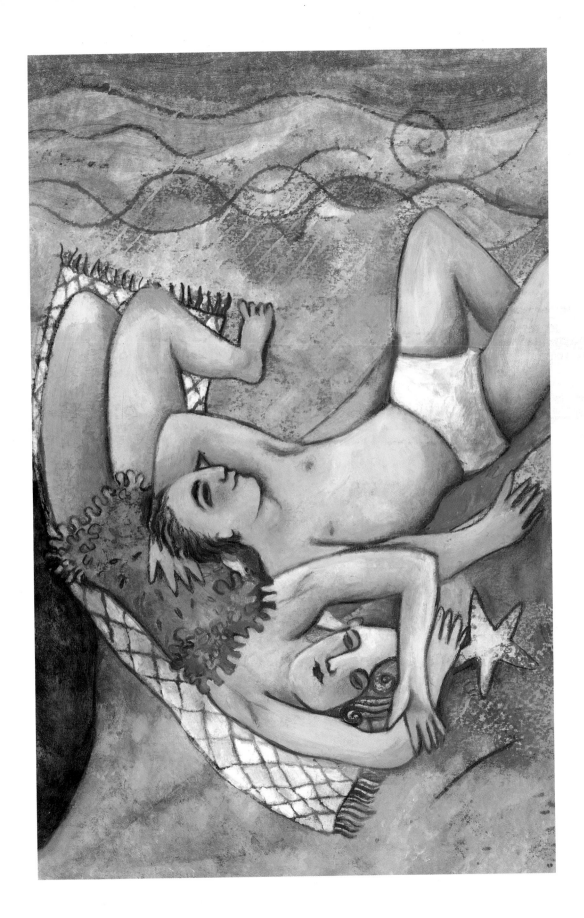

golden sand; in front of you the sea is a wonderful blue; behind you there are sand dunes, trees and a grassy bank; above you the sky is a beautiful light blue with only a few scattered, fluffy white clouds breaking up the blue.

The beach is almost deserted. To your left you can just hear the sound of children playing. To your right you can vaguely hear voices. Out on the water there are one or two cries of laughter and joy from a group of swimmers splashing in the shallow waters.

The most insistent sound you can hear is that of the sea breaking on the shore. It has a rhythmic, comforting sound which makes you feel sleepy.

High, high above the sun is shining and you can feel its warmth on your skin. Your feet and legs are warm. Your tummy is warm. Your chest and arms are warm. And you can feel the warmth of the sun on your face. Your eyelids are closed and the warmth, too, is helping to make you feel sleepy and very relaxed.

Although you are lying comfortably on the beach allow your spirit to float upwards for a moment or two; look down at yourself from high up in the sky.

You are dressed in just a bathing costume and you look strong, fit, slim and healthy. You suddenly realize that you are now as slim as you always wanted to be. You look wonderful.

All around you the sand is golden. Behind you the grassy bank is a glorious green. In front of you the white breakers of the sea collapse and die on the sand with relentless monotony. You watch yourself moving about on your beach towel and you suddenly realise that there are no signs of arthritis. There are no signs of any stiffness and you do not seem to be in any pain. You look strong, healthy and slim and you feel proud of your body.

*"If you have been ignoring your health for years it will take you a while to learn how to listen to it again – but if you persevere then you will succeed ."*

As you look down at yourself you realize that you achieved this success by eating only when you were hungry; by never eating because you were depressed or bored. You realize too that you were strong enough not to eat when you were no longer hungry and you feel proud of yourself for your willpower.

You have a wonderful figure and you look healthy. You are proud of yourself. You see yourself as a success. You know that you follow a very simple rule: if you aren't hungry you don't eat. You realize that this is the simple secret of constant slimming success.

You look down at yourself for one last time and then you drift downwards and back into your body.

Back down on the beach you can feel the warmth of the sun on your face, your chest and your arms, your stomach, your legs and your feet; you can hear the sound of the waves breaking on the shore.

Slowly, you open your eyes and you wake up. And your determination to succeed is stronger than ever. You know that you can lose your unwanted weight and you know that this will help to keep your arthritis under control.

---

**WARNING**
**Never play your slimming tape when you are driving or operating machinery as it may make you feel drowsy.**

---

## CASE HISTORY

Enid had suffered from osteoarthritis for seven years and during that time she had steadily put on weight. When I first saw her she weighed 56 lb (25 kg) more than she should have done and she found walking so difficult and so painful that she rarely moved out of her home.

She looked 10 years older than she was. In the mornings she would lie in bed until her husband helped her up. Then she would spend most of the day sitting in a comfortable chair by the fire. Because she did not go out she lost interest in her appearance and she let herself go. She never bothered with her hair, she never wore make up and she invariably wore the same colourless, shapeless and rather grubby clothes.

Inevitably, because she was bored, she spent much of her time eating. And because she took very little exercise to burn up the calories which she was consuming she steadily put on weight. Her life seemed to have become a vicious circle: her osteoarthritis made it difficult for her to move; she ate more than her body needed; she put on weight; and as she put on the extra weight so she found movement more painful.

I persuaded Enid to try to lose weight and I gave her a copy of my Slimming Tape to help boost her willpower.

The result may not have been dramatic but the diet certainly worked!

Within a mere month Enid had lost over 7 lb (3.1 kg) and within three months she had lost 28 (12.6 kg)! Most important of all, she had lost this weight not by going on a short-term diet but by changing her eating habits for good.

To her delight she found that without the excess weight to carry around she could walk far more easily. Her osteoarthritis had not changed but without so much excess weight to carry her joints were far less painful when she walked.

Today Enid is unrecognizable. She looks ten years younger than her real age. She and her husband go out together several evenings a week and occasionally she has even tried a little old-fashioned ballroom dancing.

Dieting has changed Enid's life!

## GIVE UP EATING MEAT

A vegetarian diet does seem to help arthritis – though whether it helps non-inflammatory types of arthritis such as osteoarthritis as much as it seems to help inflammation disorders such as rheumatoid arthritis is open to question. You will find advice on how to follow a vegetarian diet on pages 82–8.

## LEARN TO RELAX

When muscles are tightened and tensed by stress, joints will suffer more than when muscles are loose and relaxed. Loosen your muscles by following the relaxation exercises on pages 33–5.

## LEARN HOW TO DEAL WITH PAIN

Pain is the single most important symptom associated with osteoarthritis. Although drugs such as aspirin can be extremely effective in helping to combat pain there are many other techniques for controlling it. The most effective are described on pages 68–81.

## EXERCISE WHENEVER YOU CAN

Regular exercise will help to keep joints loose and supple. If you spend too long keeping still in order to prevent discomfort you will find that your joints are much worse when you eventually have to move. Combating osteoarthritis is a compromise: when your joints are sore or painful and when movement hurts you should rest, but when you can move you should. A regular exercise programme should push all your joints (including those not yet affected by the disease) through a full range of movements.

## BUILD UP YOUR SELF CONFIDENCE

Sufferers from osteoarthritis are, like sufferers from rheumatoid arthritis, apt to lack self-confidence. Build up self-confidence by reading the advice given on pages 38–40.

## LEARN TO LET YOUR FEELINGS SHOW

Holding in anger and sadness will make your osteoarthritis far worse. You will benefit enormously if you can let your emotions show. Read the advice on pages 40–2.

# TWENTY-FIVE TOP SLIMMING TIPS

1. NEVER EAT UP OTHER PEOPLE'S LEFTOVERS. MANY WOULD-BE SLIMMERS HATE THROWING FOOD AWAY – BUT BY EATING UP OTHER PEOPLE'S LEFTOVER FOOD YOU ARE TURNING YOURSELF INTO A DUSTBIN. IS THAT REALLY THE WAY YOU WANT TO SEE YOURSELF?

2. TRY TO EAT SNACKS INSTEAD OF MAIN MEALS. IF YOU EAT FIVE OR SIX SMALL MEALS – INSTEAD OF TWO OR THREE LARGE ONES – YOU WILL FIND IT EASIER TO EAT THE AMOUNT OF FOOD THAT YOUR BODY REALLY NEEDS.

3. WAIT FOR FIVE MINUTES WHENEVER YOU FEEL THAT YOU WANT TO EAT SOMETHING. BY THEN THE URGE TO EAT MAY HAVE GONE.

4. WHEN YOU EAT CONCENTRATE ON WHAT YOU ARE DOING – YOU WILL BE MORE LIKELY TO HEAR YOUR BODY TELLING YOU THAT YOU ARE FULL.

5. REGULAR EXERCISE WILL HELP TO BURN UP UNNEEDED CALORIES AND IT WILL ALSO HELP TO TONE UP YOUR MUSCLES.

6. TRY TO RELAX BEFORE YOU SIT DOWN TO A MEAL. IF YOU EAT WHEN YOU ARE TENSE YOU WILL PROBABLY EAT MORE THAN YOU REALLY NEED.

7. DON'T LET OTHER PEOPLE FORCE YOU TO EAT FOOD THAT YOU NEITHER WANT NOR NEED. WHEN YOU ARE FULL DON'T BE AFRAID TO SAY SO!

8. WHENEVER YOU ARE ABOUT TO PUT FOOD INTO YOUR MOUTH ASK YOURSELF WHETHER OR NOT YOU REALLY NEED IT. IF YOU DON'T THEN DON'T EAT IT!

9. IF YOU EAT IN THE EVENING YOUR BODY WILL STORE THE UNWANTED FOOD AS FAT. IF YOU DO MOST OF YOUR EATING EARLY IN THE DAY YOUR BODY WILL BURN UP THE EXCESS CALORIES.

10. DON'T RUSH FROM ONE COURSE TO THE NEXT. TRY TO TAKE A BREAK BETWEEN COURSES.

11. WHEN YOU HAVE FINISHED EATING LEAVE THE TABLE. IF YOU STAY YOU WILL PROBABLY NIBBLE.

12. INSTEAD OF USING SUGAR BUY – AND USE – SWEETENERS.

13. WEIGH YOURSELF NO MORE THAN ONCE A WEEK WHEN YOU ARE TRYING TO LOSE WEIGHT. IF YOU WEIGH YOURSELF TOO OFTEN YOU MAY BECOME DEPRESSED WHEN YOUR WEIGHT LOSS ISN'T INSTANTLY NOTICEABLE.

14. JOIN A SLIMMING CLUB TO GET THE SUPPORT OF OTHER SLIMMERS AND ADVICE FROM EXPERIENCED TEACHERS.

15. DON'T EAT WHILE WATCHING TV – IT'S TOO EASY TO CONTINUE PUTTING FOOD INTO YOUR MOUTH WHEN YOU'RE CONCENTRATING ON SOMETHING ELSE.

16. IGNORE MAGIC DIETS PROMISING ENORMOUS AND RAPID WEIGHT LOSSES. IF YOU DON'T, YOU WILL ONLY PUT THE WEIGHT BACK ON AGAIN

17. IF YOU ARE BORED OR MISERABLE AND YOU ARE TEMPTED TO EAT TO CHEER YOURSELF UP, DON'T. GO AND BUY YOURSELF A GIFT SUCH AS A BOOK OR A BUNCH OF FLOWERS INSTEAD.

18. DON'T WASTE MONEY ON SLIMMING PILLS OR DIETARY SUPPLEMENTS.

19. TALK TO YOUR DOCTOR AND ASK FOR HIS HELP. MORE AND MORE HEALTH CARE PROFESSIONALS NOW REALIZE THE IMPORTANCE OF HELPING THEIR PATIENTS TACKLE THEIR EXCESS WEIGHT.

20. DRINK A LOW-CALORIE DRINK SUCH AS WATER, LOW-CALORIE SOUP, BLACK TEA OR COFFEE HALF-AN-HOUR BEFORE A MEAL IN ORDER TO FILL YOUR STOMACH AND REDUCE YOUR APPETITE.

21. RESIST THE TEMPTATION TO TASTE FOOD WHEN YOU ARE PREPARING IT. THIS SORT OF EATING HAS NOTHING TO DO WITH HUNGER – AND IS PROBABLY ONE OF THE REASONS WHY SO MANY PEOPLE WHO WORK IN THE CATERING INDUSTRY ARE OVERWEIGHT.

22. REMEMBER THAT YOU DON'T HAVE TO HAVE A CUP OF COFFEE AND A BISCUIT JUST BECAUSE IT IS BREAK-TIME. INSTEAD OF EATING WHY NOT READ A MAGAZINE, WRITE A LETTER OR MAKE A TELEPHONE CALL?

23. WHEN YOU HAVE LOST WEIGHT, THROW OUT THE CLOTHES THAT NO LONGER FIT YOU. IF YOU KEEP THEM THEN YOU ARE ADMITTING THAT YOU DO NOT EXPECT YOUR WEIGHT LOSS TO BE PERMANENT.

24. MANY PRESCRIBED PILLS, SUCH AS STEROIDS, CAN PRODUCE WEIGHT GAIN. IF YOU ARE TAKING ANY PRESCRIBED DRUG TALK TO YOUR DOCTOR AND ASK HIM IF HE THINKS IT COULD AFFECT YOUR ABILITY TO LOSE WEIGHT. THERE MAY BE AN ALTERNATIVE DRUG.

25. RICE IS AN EXCELLENT FOOD – SO EAT MORE OF IT. IT'S FILLING, FULL OF NOURISHMENT AND LOW IN CALORIES. PASTA, TOO, IS ANOTHER UNDERUSED FOOD IN MANY HOMES.

# Height / Weight Chart for Women

| Height | | Ideal Weight Band | |
| IMPERIAL (Feet/Inches) | METRIC (Metres) | IMPERIAL (Stones /Pounds) | METRIC (Kilograms) |
| --- | --- | --- | --- |
| 4.10 | 1.47 | 7.5 – 8.5 | 46.7 – 53.0 |
| 4.11 | 1.49 | 7.7 – 8.7 | 47.6 – 53.9 |
| 5.0 | 1.52 | 7.9 – 8.9 | 48.5 – 54.8 |
| 5.1 | 1.54 | 7.11 – 8.11 | 49.4 – 55.7 |
| 5.2 | 1.57 | 8.1 – 9.1 | 51.2 – 57.6 |
| 5.3 | 1.60 | 8.4 – 9.4 | 52.6 – 58.9 |
| 5.4 | 1.62 | 8.6 – 9.6 | 53.5 – 59.8 |
| 5.5 | 1.65 | 8.10 – 9.10 | 55.3 – 61.6 |
| 5.6 | 1.67 | 9.0 – 10.0 | 57.0 – 63.5 |
| 5.7 | 1.70 | 9.3 – 10.3 | 58.5 – 64.8 |
| 5.8 | 1.72 | 9.7 – 10.7 | 60.0 – 66.6 |
| 5.9 | 1.75 | 9.10 – 10.10 | 61.6 – 68.0 |
| 5.10 | 1.77 | 10.0 – 11.0 | 63.5 – 69.8 |
| 5.11 | 1.80 | 10.3 – 11.3 | 64.8 – 71.2 |
| 6.0 | 1.82 | 10.7 – 11.7 | 66.6 – 73.0 |
| 6.1 | 1.85 | 10.9 – 11.9 | 67.5 – 73.9 |
| 6.2 | 1.87 | 10.12 – 11.12 | 68.9 – 75.2 |
| 6.3 | 1.90 | 11.2 – 12.2 | 70.7 – 77.1 |
| 6.4 | 1.93 | 11.5 – 12.5 | 72.1 – 78.4 |

## Instructions

1. Weigh yourself with as few clothes as possible – and no shoes.
2. Measure your height in bare or stockinged feet
3. You are overweight if your weight falls above your ideal weight band

Note: Ideal weights vary with age and various other factors, but if you weigh more than 14 lb (6.3 kg) above the maximum in your Ideal Weight Band then your weight will almost certainly be having an adverse effect on your joints.

# Height / Weight Chart for Men

| HEIGHT | | IDEAL WEIGHT BAND | |
|---|---|---|---|
| IMPERIAL | METRIC | IMPERIAL | METRIC |
| (FEET/INCHES) | (METRES) | (STONES /POUNDS) | (KILOGRAMS) |
| 5.0 | 1.52 | 8.5 – 9.5 | 53.0 – 59.4 |
| 5.1 | 1.54 | 8.6 – 9.6 | 53.5 – 59.8 |
| 5.2 | 1.57 | 8.7 – 9.7 | 53.9 – 60.0 |
| 5.3 | 1.60 | 8.8 – 9.8 | 54.4 – 60.7 |
| 5.4 | 1.62 | 8.11 – 9.11 | 55.7 – 62.1 |
| 5.5 | 1.65 | 9.2 – 10.2 | 58.0 – 64.4 |
| 5.6 | 1.67 | 9.6 – 10.6 | 59.8 – 66.2 |
| 5.7 | 1.70 | 9.10 – 10.10 | 61.6 – 68.0 |
| 5.8 | 1.72 | 10.0 –11.0 | 63.5 – 69.8 |
| 5.9 | 1.75 | 10.4 – 11.4 | 65.3 – 71.6 |
| 5.10 | 1.77 | 10.8 – 11.8 | 61.7 – 73.4 |
| 5.11 | 1.80 | 10.12 – 11.12 | 68.9 – 75.2 |
| 6.0 | 1.82 | 11.2 – 12.2 | 70.7 – 77.1 |
| 6.1 | 1.85 | 11.6 – 12.6 | 72.5 – 78.9 |
| 6.2 | 1.87 | 11.10 – 12.10 | 74.3 – 80.7 |
| 6.3 | 1.90 | 12.0 – 13.0 | 76.2 – 82.5 |
| 6.4 | 1.93 | 12.4 – 13.4 | 78.0 – 84.3 |
| 6.5 | 1.95 | 12.8 – 13.8 | 79.8 – 86.1 |
| 6.6 | 1.98 | 13.0 – 14.0 | 82.5 – 88.9 |

## INSTRUCTIONS

1. Weigh yourself with as few clothes as possible – and no shoes
2. Measure your height in bare or stockinged feet
3. You are overweight if your weight falls above your ideal weight band

Note: Ideal weights vary with age and various other factors, but if you weigh more than 14 lb (6.3 kg) above the maximum in your Ideal Weight Band then your weight will almost certainly be having an adverse effect on your joints.

# CHAPTER FOUR

# Other Arthritic Disorders

*Rheumatoid arthritis and osteoarthritis are, without a doubt, the two most common and most important arthritic disorders. However, they are not the only arthritic disorders. This chapter describes the most common and most important of the other arthritic disorders.*

## TREATMENTS

Many of the treatment techniques described in Chapters Two and Three of this book are effective in the control of these disorders. Please talk to your own doctor and ask for advice about which treatments will be most useful for you.

## ANKYLOSING SPONDYLITIS

### WHICH ARE THE JOINTS INVOLVED?

The joints of the spine, particularly the lower back, are most commonly affected but sometimes the larger joints of the body also become inflamed and stiff. 'Spondylitis' means inflammation of the spine and 'ankylosing' means stiffening. Although the disease tends to start at the bottom of the spine it usually travels upwards over the years.

### WHO GETS ANKYLOSING SPONDYLITIS?

The most common sufferers are young white males between the ages of 15 and 25–but women can be affected as well. Ankylosing spondylitis tends to run in families. It affects between 1 in 200 and 1 in 400 people.

### WHAT CAUSES ANKYLOSING SPONDYLITIS?

The stiffness is caused by an inflammation where the ligaments are attached to bones but just what causes this inflammation is still a mystery.

Ankylosing spondylitis may be inherited (it is definitely associated with a particular gene) and may be caused by an infection or some other environmental factor. It is quite different to rheumatoid arthritis (another inflammatory disorder). In rheumatoid arthritis the inflammation is inside the joints. In ankylosing spondylitis the inflammation affects the edges of the joints. As time goes by the inflamed joint edges turn into bone, and it is this that causes the stiffness. Eventually, the new bone may join two vertebrae together completely so that part of the back becomes rigid.

### WHAT ARE THE SYMPTOMS?

Pain and stiffness in the back and any other joints involved are the first and most obvious symptoms that a sufferer will notice. If a nerve is trapped there may be pain going down the back of the leg. These symptoms are usually worse in the mornings and after resting and they are relieved by exercise. The symptoms gradually get worse and worse as time goes by, with the patient becoming stiffer and stiffer and finding the act of bending increasingly difficult. There is also sometimes inflammation of the eye(s), the skin and of other parts of the body. Ankylosing spondylitis tends to burn itself out at around the age of 50 or so as the inflammation becomes less intense.

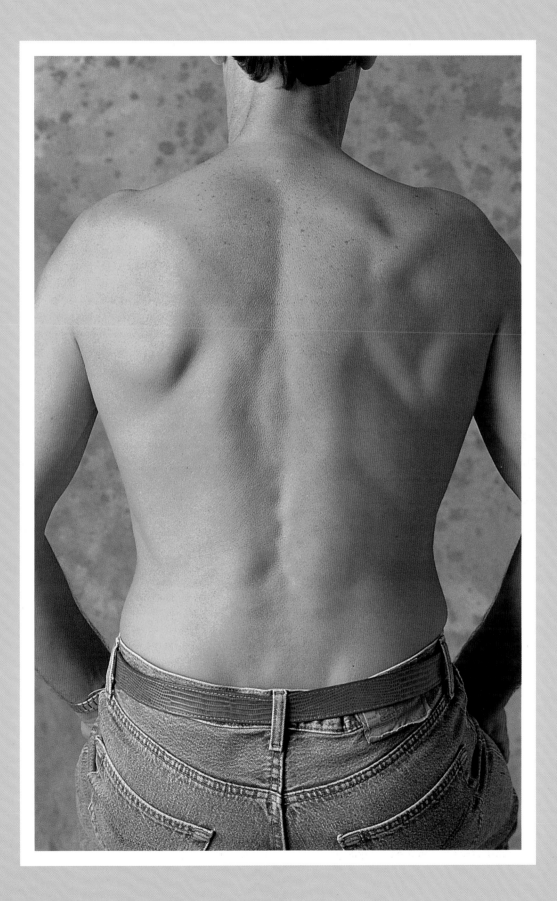

### TREATMENT

Regular exercise is vitally important since it can help to delay stiffening of the spine. For the same reason physiotherapy is also important. Drugs normally used in the treatment of rheumatoid arthritis and osteoarthritis are sometimes used to help control the pain and stiffness associated with ankylosing spondylitis.

## GOUT

### WHICH JOINTS ARE INVOLVED?

Any joint in the body can be affected but the big toes are the ones most commonly involved. The ankles, knees, wrists, elbows and fingers are also common sites for gout.

### WHO GETS GOUT?

Gout is fairly common and affects men rather than women (in a ratio of 20 to 1). Gout usually affects individuals between the ages of 35 and 60 and it runs in families. Most gout sufferers are rather overweight and often also have high blood pressure. However, many sufferers only get one or two attacks a year.

### WHAT CAUSES GOUT?

Gout develops when the levels of uric acid in the blood get too high and uric acid crystals accumulate in the joints, where they may eventually cause damage. Normally, uric acid is formed when waste products are broken down in the body. In a healthy individual the uric acid is excreted in the urine but gout sufferers fail to get rid of all the uric acid their bodies are making. There are several possible reasons for this. The kidneys may be damaged, and therefore not expelling uric acid properly. There may be an inherited tendency to high levels of uric acid. Alternatively the problem may simply be caused by eating too many foods which are broken down to produce high levels of uric acid. Prescribed drugs can sometimes trigger a high uric acid level and an attack of gout.

### WHAT ARE THE SYMPTOMS?

Gout usually begins with a fairly sudden onset of severe pain in a joint which is usually swollen and rather bluish red in colour. There may also be a moderate fever. The symptoms of gout tend to come and go quite unexpectedly. The first attack usually begins with an itchy, swollen toe which gradually becomes painful. If gout is untreated it may eventually lead to joint damage, producing long-term symptoms rather similar to those associated with osteoarthritis.

### TREATMENT

Patients with acute gout are usually advised to rest. Anti-inflammatory drugs are sometimes prescribed to ease pain and some patients need long-term treatment with drugs which prevent the accumulation of uric acid or aid the kidneys to get rid of uric acid, thereby helping to prevent pain recurring. Many patients notice an improvement in their condition if they lose weight and avoid certain foods or drugs. Foods which are particularly likely to cause problems include: meat extracts, game, asparagus, spinach, strawberries, rhubarb, fish roe, herring, salmon, whitebait,

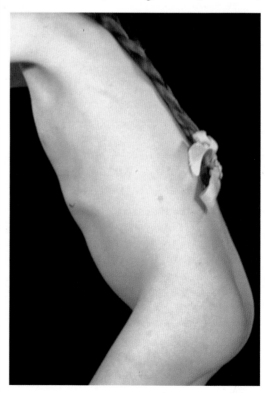

*Juvenile rheumatoid arthritis*

liver, kidneys and sweetbreads. Drinks which can cause gout include: carbonated drinks, beer, sparkling wines, port, champagne and many other kinds of alcohol. Treatment of gout is important because if uric acid levels are allowed to remain high the kidneys may be damaged by an accumulation of crystals.

## JUVENILE RHEUMATOID ARTHRITIS

### WHICH JOINTS ARE INVOLVED?

There are several different types of juvenile rheumatoid arthritis but overall the small joints of the fingers, toes, wrists and ankles are the ones most commonly affected. The neck, shoulders, hips and knees may also be involved.

### WHO GETS JUVENILE RHEUMATOID ARTHRITIS?

Children of any age can be affected but juvenile arthritis affects girls more often than boys. It most commonly starts either very early (between the ages of two and four) or just before or around puberty. It is not a common disease.

### WHAT CAUSES JUVENILE RHEUMATOID ARTHRITIS?

Very little is known about its cause although it does appear to be inherited.

### WHAT ARE THE SYMPTOMS?

The illness usually begins with a high fever and most sufferers start feeling unwell before any joint problems appear. Children with juvenile rheumatoid arthritis may fail to grow properly, may lose weight and may complain of abdominal pains. The heart, liver, spleen and lymph nodes may be affected, the eyes may be inflamed and there may be a skin rash. Joint symptoms may not start until the disease has been present for some months.

### TREATMENT

Three-quarters of sufferers from juvenile rheumatoid arthritis recover completely. Careful exercise, the splinting of affected joints to protect them,

physiotherapy and rest all help. Children are usually advised to avoid contact sports which might result in joint injury. Both drugs and surgery are sometimes used.

## POLYMYALGIA RHEUMATICA

### WHICH JOINTS ARE INVOLVED?

The hips, shoulders, thighs and neck are most commonly affected.

### WHO GETS POLYMYALGIA RHEUMATICA?

Polymyalgia rheumatica affects two or three times as many women as men. It doesn't usually affect anyone under the age of 50. It is uncommon.

### WHAT CAUSES POLYMYALGIA RHEUMATICA?

The cause of the pain and discomfort associated with polymyalgia rheumatica is unknown.

### WHAT ARE THE SYMPTOMS?

The main symptoms of polymyalgia rheumatica are tenderness and discomfort in the hips, shoulders and neck. The discomfort is at its worst early on in the morning, gradually getting worse again later on in the day. Many patients have difficulty in getting out of bed, also often complaining of depression, tiredness, weakness, weight loss and fever. This may develop gradually or suddenly.

### TREATMENT

Steroids usually provide dramatic relief. Indeed, the results are so spectacular that giving steroids is sometimes regarded as a diagnostic test for this disease. A carefully balanced course of steroid treatment may be necessary for some time. (See dangers of steroid treatment on pages 25–6).

## PSORIATIC ARTHRITIS

### WHICH JOINTS ARE INVOLVED?

Psoriasis is a fairly common skin disease in which patches of skin become inflamed, red and scaly. Psoriatic arthritis can affect any joint in the body but is usually restricted to just one or two joints.

The joints near to the finger tips are particularly likely to be affected.

## WHO GETS PSORIATIC ARTHRITIS?

Psoriatic arthritis affects one in ten psoriasis sufferers. Psoriasis affects approximately one in 50 people; one in ten of those get psoriatic arthritis.

## WHAT CAUSES PSORIATIC ARTHRITIS?

No one really understands the link between psoriasis and arthritis (although there are lots of theories). It seems likely, however, that both skin and joints are affected by inflammation.

## WHAT ARE THE SYMPTOMS?

The symptoms depend upon the type of arthritis that develops. Some patients develop symptoms similar to rheumatoid arthritis (although the symptoms tend to be less severe). Others get ankylosing spondylitis. Individual joints – particularly those in the fingers and toes – may be affected or the disease may flare up intermittently in different joints around the body. Psoriatic

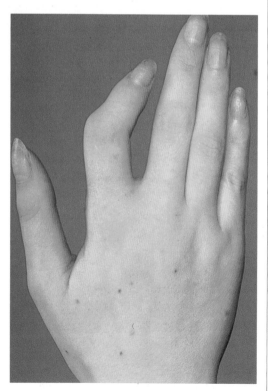

*Psoriatic arthritis affects finger joints.*

arthritis tends to be even more unpredictable than the other forms of arthritis.

## TREATMENT

The treatment of the joint symptoms will depend upon the type of arthritis involved. Usually skin and joint problems are treated separately because the powerful drugs which can treat both problems simultaneously are very likely to produce unpleasant side effects.

## REACTIVE ARTHRITIS

### WHICH JOINTS ARE INVOLVED?

The joints of the legs – knees, ankles and feet – are affected more commonly than any other.

### WHO GETS REACTIVE ARTHRITIS?

Men are affected more than women and young adults (between 18 and 35) are the group most likely to suffer from reactive arthritis. The disease is not very common.

### WHAT CAUSES REACTIVE ARTHRITIS?

Reactive arthritis is triggered by an infection of the bowel or urinary tract. Sometimes the trigger is a sexually transmitted infection.

### WHAT ARE THE SYMPTOMS?

The joints affected are likely to develop arthritic symptoms and in addition there is likely to be an inflammation of the eyes, skin and mouth. Patients usually complain of sore eyes, skin rashes, pain on passing urine and mouth ulcers as well as the joint symptoms.

### TREATMENT

Treatment will depend very much on the symptoms. The infection which has caused the generalized inflammation will probably need treating first of all but if the joints are badly affected anti-inflammatory drugs may be needed. If fluid has accumulated in the joints some of it may need to be drawn off. Painful joints may need rest. Reactive arthritis does not usually produce any long-term damage.

# RHEUMATIC FEVER

## WHICH JOINTS ARE INVOLVED?

Rheumatic fever affects large joints such as the knees but moves from joint to joint rarely affecting any one joint for more than a few days.

## WHO GETS RHEUMATIC FEVER?

The disease affects children between the ages of 5 and 15. It is rare in the developed countries but still common in Asia and Africa.

## WHAT CAUSES RHEUMATIC FEVER?

It starts as a throat infection which triggers an immune response. Experts believe that rheumatic fever can be prevented by treating throat infections promptly with antibiotics.

## WHAT ARE THE SYMPTOMS?

Patients usually complain of a persistent fever and pains which flit from joint to joint. As soon as one joint recovers another becomes affected. The joints are swollen, painful and hot. There is usually a sore throat two weeks before joint pains start. These symptoms normally last a few weeks. The most dangerous aspect is that about half of all patients develop heart trouble, though the damage may not become apparent for several years. It may also cause a skin rash and small lumps in the skin. If the nervous system is affected uncontrollable, jerky movements may develop.

## TREATMENT

Rest is vitally important. Penicillin is normally needed to deal with the infection. Aspirin is the most effective pain-killer. If the heart valves are affected heart surgery may be needed later on.

# RHEUMATISM

This is a word which is used to describe most aches or pains affecting a bone, joint or muscle.

# SEPTIC ARTHRITIS

## WHICH JOINTS ARE INVOLVED?

Any joint can be affected by septic arthritis – it attacks the body indiscriminately.

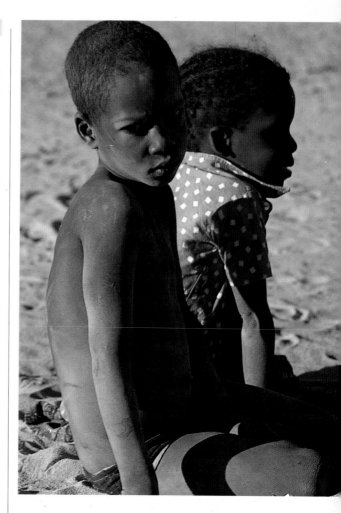

*Rheumatic fever is common in Africa.*

## WHO GETS SEPTIC ARTHRITIS?

It can affect anyone but sufferers of rheumatoid arthritis or diabetes are particularly susceptible.

## WHAT CAUSES SEPTIC ARTHRITIS?

A variety of organisms, injections into a joint or surgery on or around a joint. Steroid treatment makes septic arthritis more likely.

## WHAT ARE THE SYMPTOMS?

The main symptoms are a sudden onset of swelling, heat and tenderness in joints, limited joint movement and a fever.

## TREATMENT

Antibiotics are usually needed and the joint may need to be drained.

# CHAPTER FIVE

# The Control Of Pain

*Whatever sort of arthritis you suffer from, pain is more likely to cause misery, unhappiness and despair than all your other symptoms put together. Left untreated, or badly treated, pain leads to physical and mental exhaustion, disablement and chronic depression. Patients with persistent pain need to spend long periods in bed and are far more likely to develop other serious medical complications. They get better more slowly and need more support from friends, family and professionals.*

## THE CONQUERING OF PAIN

Everyone suffers from pain some of the time. Some people suffer from pain most of the time. And thousands of very unlucky people suffer from pain all of the time.

Pain is the one symptom just about all arthritis sufferers hate, fear and complain about – but it is one symptom that doctors are terrible at treating. Most doctors know very little about pain control. Many medical textbooks dismiss pain as though it were an irrelevance, and medical schools do not bother to teach students much about pain relief.

Worst of all, there seems to be a conspiracy between doctors and drug companies which ensures that millions of patients in pain are denied easy, cheap, reliable pain relief so that profits can remain high.

You think I'm exaggerating? Read on.

## THE GATE CONTROL THEORY

The story began when what is called 'the gate control' theory of pain was accepted.

The gate control theory, put forward by two scientists called Melzack and Wall, suggested that when body tissues are damaged messages carrying information about the injury travel towards the brain along two quite separate sets of nerve fibres.

The larger fibres carry messages about sensations other than pain and the smaller fibres carry the pain messages. The messages which travel along the larger fibres tend to arrive at the spinal cord before the messages travelling along the smaller fibres and, if there are enough non-painful sensations travelling, the pain messages won't be able to get through.

Once this theory had been accepted it was possible to explain all sorts of natural phenomena which had, up until then, been a mystery.

For example, it became clear that when we rub a sore spot what we are doing is increasing the number of non-pain messages travelling towards the spinal cord (and thence the brain). If you knock your elbow you will automatically reach to rub the spot because subconsciously you know that by rubbing the area you will be able to cut down the amount of pain that you feel.

## THE TENS MACHINE

Once it was discovered just how rubbing a sore or painful place can relieve pain the next step was to come up with a way of stimulating the passage of non-painful sensations even more efficiently – and doctors came up with the idea of using electricity to produce the necessary stimulus.

As a result of various experiments it was

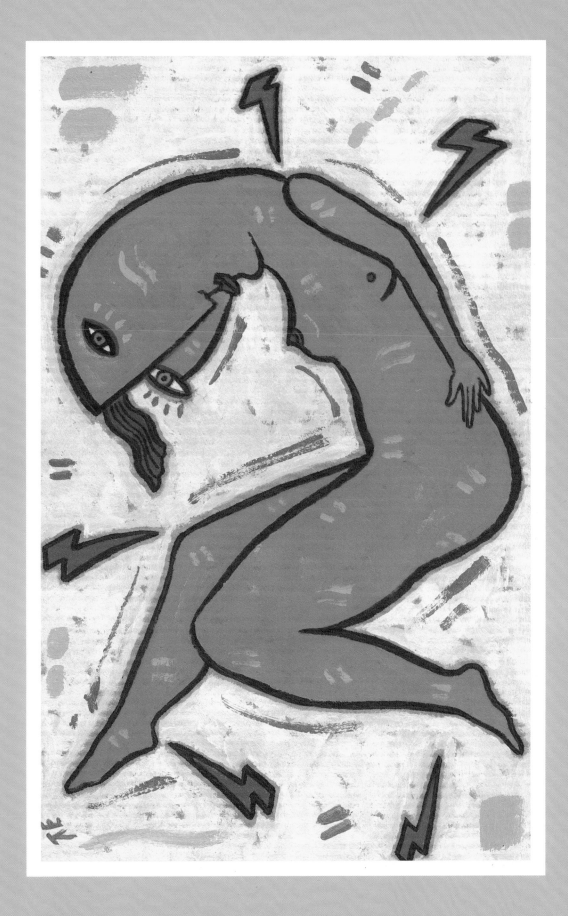

discovered that by giving patients small pocket-sized devices that sent out a series of electrical pulses, the passage of pain messages could be successfully blocked.

The technique was called Transcutaneous Electrical Nerve Stimulation and the devices which were used were called TENS machines. It was quickly found that in addition to sending sensory messages which blocked the passage of pain impulses the TENS machines also encouraged the body to produce its own endorphins or pain-relieving hormones.

Numerous studies have shown that patients with disorders such as arthritis can benefit enormously from using TENS machines. There are very few side effects and the machines cost relatively little to buy (compared to the cost of a year's supply of pain-killers they are a very good buy).

If you want to try a TENS machine talk to your own doctor. Although many members of the medical profession are still unaware of the existence or usefulness of TENS machines (largely because the majority of doctors still get most of their post-graduate education from drug companies which obviously have a vested interest in not telling doctors about devices which could destroy the multi-million pound analgesic industry), a growing number are learning about them. If your own doctor has never heard of these extremely effective devices ask him or her to arrange for you to see a consultant at your local hospital or, alternatively, ask him or her for a referral to the nearest specialist pain clinic.

## KNOW WHEN AND HOW TO REST

It is a mistake to rest too much. If you suffer regularly from sore or painful joints you should try to keep as active as you possibly can and try to

*"If you suffer regularly from sore or painful joints you should try to keep as active as you possibly can and try to move your joints whenever they are not painful."*

move your joints whenever they are not painful.

The danger is that if you rest too much both your body and your mind will stagnate; your muscles will become weak and flabby (so you will run a greater risk than usual of falling when you do try to move about) and your mind will slow down.

But, having said all that, there is absolutely no doubt that there are times when rest is important – and, as an arthritis sufferer, it is vitally important that you know when and how to rest.

First, the 'when'. You must learn to recognize when your body really needs rest, and when too much activity will make your pain worse rather than better.

The most important thing to remember is that whenever you have an acute or sudden attack of pain you should make sure that you rest. Do not try to be brave or be a 'hero', for if you do the chances are that you will damage your joints even more. You should always avoid doing anything that makes your pain more severe or that seems to make your condition worse in any other way.

This does not, however, mean that you should never move any part of your body that feels uncomfortable. Many arthritis sufferers are never really free of discomfort. It is vital to keep moving those joints which are sore for if you do not move them there is a real danger that they will deteriorate even further. You should try to differentiate between genuine and threatening pain (which means that you should rest as much as you can) and modest and bearable discomfort (when you can move without creating extra pain).

You should also be prepared to rest whenever you feel tired. Some arthritis sufferers who have heard that patients who do not move will become 'fixed' in one position and permanently disabled are so determined to keep mobile and active that they force themselves to keep moving all the time

– even when they are completely exhausted.

While it is important to keep active and busy, if you try to force your body to do too much by pushing yourself more and more you will exhaust your reserves and you will, ironically, increase your susceptibility to pain. It is vitally important that you learn to recognize your limits. You must be prepared to take a break when you feel that your body needs a rest – if you attempt to fight your body's demands you will find that you lose far more time in recovering from the damage you have inflicted upon yourself.

In addition to learning WHEN to rest you must also learn HOW to rest so that your body gets the full benefit.

For example, it is extremely important that you do not succumb to the temptation to put pillows under sore joints to ease them and to hold uncomfortable limbs in fixed positions. There is a real risk that if you do this then your joints will become immobilized in an entirely impractical and very difficult position. Always bear it in mind that painful joints can stiffen up very quickly indeed.

As well as taking short breaks when your joints are stiff and painful you should also try to make sure that you take more long-term breaks when you can.

Like everyone else, arthritis patients are vulnerable to stress and pressure and when they are exposed to problems their general health will usually suffer – and, inevitably, their joints will become more painful.

Consequently, taking regular breaks away from your everyday stresses and worries is a very important part of your treatment and pain control programme. You don't have to go anywhere expensive, of course – these days it can often be cheaper to spend a few days out of season at the seaside (perhaps even on the shores of the Mediterranean) than it is to stay at home.

Try to make sure that you go somewhere peaceful and relaxing where you can unwind and escape from pressure. Remember that if your body needs a break then your mind does too.

## WHAT AFFECTS YOUR PAIN THRESHOLD?

Everyone has their own personal pain threshold, which is the level of pain which has to be reached before it is felt and recognized by your body as pain. Your tissues will only produce the chemical necessary to stimulate a nervous response and send pain messages to your brain if you have inflicted a certain amount of damage.

If, for example, you scratch yourself on a bramble in the garden you may not even notice it has happened and you probably won't think of the sensation you feel as pain. If, on the other hand, you cut your finger with a kitchen knife

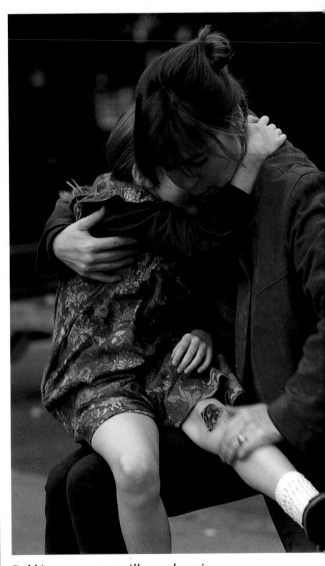

*Rubbing a sore spot will ease the pain.*

while chopping vegetables you are quite likely to feel what you would describe as pain.

Pain thresholds vary from one individual to another. But, more important still, your pain threshold varies from minute to minute according to a variety of factors which you may find surprising. Here are some of them:

### HOW DISTRACTED YOU ARE

If your mind is busily occupied with something else you may not even notice you are in pain and your pain threshold will also be much higher. Experiments have shown that volunteers found that they could put up with extra pain if they listened to music they liked or if they were shown pictures to distract them.

### HOW FRIGHTENED YOU ARE

If you believe the pain you feel signifies a serious illness or injury you are likely to suffer more from the pain. Fear of the unknown lowers your pain threshold and your pain tolerance level (your pain tolerance level is the amount of pain you can stand). However, by the time you have seen your doctor and been reassured that your headache doesn't mean you have a brain tumour or that your stomach ache isn't appendicitis you will feel less anxious. You will walk out of the doctor's surgery feeling confident and suffering less from your pain with every step.

### WHETHER YOU ARE DEPRESSED

Your response to pain is influenced by your mood, so if you are feeling unhappy and you cut your finger then the pain will seem worse than if you had been feeling happy.

### YOUR FAMILY CIRCUMSTANCES

If you grew up with lots of brothers and sisters you are likely to have much higher pain tolerance levels than people who grow up with fewer siblings. Only children are the most likely to have low pain thresholds and pain tolerance levels.

If you were one of several children it is likely that your parents had less time to give you individual attention and make a fuss every time you got a knock or a bruise. If you weren't fussed over you will probably have a higher pain tolerance level than a child whose parents came running whenever she complained of the tiniest scratch.

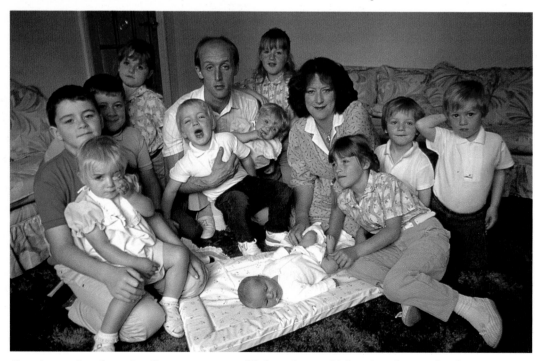

*Growing up in a large family means you are likely to have a high pain tolerance level*

# How To Measure Your Pain

IT IS IMPOSSIBLE TO MEASURE PAIN OBJECTIVELY. THERE ARE SO MANY DIFFERENT FACTORS INVOLVED THAT YOU CANNOT COMPARE THE PAIN YOU GET IN YOUR JOINTS WITH THE PAIN YOUR NEIGHBOUR GETS IN HER WOMB. HOWEVER, YOU CAN MEASURE VARIATIONS IN A PARTICULAR PAIN, AND BY DOING THIS YOU CAN TELL WHETHER OR NOT A PAIN-RELIEVING TECHNIQUE THAT YOU ARE USING IS WORKING.

Look through the list of words which follow and pick out the four which you think describe your pain most accurately:

SORE (1)   DULL (1)

TENDER (1)   ANNOYING (1)

TROUBLESOME (1)   UNCOMFORTABLE (1)

TIRING (2)   HURTING (2)

HEAVY (2)   DISTRESSING (2)

MISERABLE (2)   SICKENING (2)

EXHAUSTING (3)   FRIGHTFUL (3)

WRETCHED (3)   INTENSE (3)

HORRIBLE (3)   PUNISHING (3)

TERRIFYING (4)   VICIOUS (4)

KILLING (4)   UNBEARABLE (4)

EXCRUCIATING (4)   INTOLERABLE (4)

Add up the numbers that follow each of the four words you have chosen. The total is your PAIN SCORE.

NEXT TIME YOU WANT TO MEASURE YOUR PAIN, LOOK THROUGH THE LIST AGAIN AND REPEAT THE PROCEDURE, COMPARING YOUR TOTAL SCORE WITH PREVIOUS TOTAL SCORES.

## YOUR AGE

Your pain tolerance will change as you get older. You will become better able to tolerate superficial pains and less able to tolerate deep pains.

## HOW TO DOMINATE YOUR PAIN

Anyone who suffers from constant (or near constant) pain will confirm that before long the pain begins to take over. Many arthritis sufferers have told me that their pains and infirmities have come to rule their lives and their relationships with other people.

'It all started quite innocuously,' said one arthritis victim. 'When I first began suffering from bad arthritis my wife was very kind and understanding. She made a fuss of me and looked after me and gradually started to do more and more things for me. She fetched things for me. If I dropped the paper she picked it up for me. If I wanted some pipe tobacco she walked to the corner shop and I let her. I let her because it was quicker for her to do things and I didn't have to make any effort. But eventually I realized that our relationship had changed. Instead of treating me like a partner she was treating me like a child. By then our relationship had changed permanently. In the end my arthritis ruined my marriage and resulted in my divorce.'

If you suffer from bad arthritis and you find it difficult to get about you will almost certainly find that the people who are close to you will want to help you. Friends and relatives will make you a cup of coffee, change the television channel for you, help tie your shoe laces and so on. They do all these things out of kindness and if the pain is really bad – and you genuinely cannot move – then you will undoubtedly welcome their help with grateful thanks. But if you allow people to look after you

*"Try to regard your arthritis and the pain it brings as an enemy that can be controlled even if it cannot be conquered or banished completely'.'*

like this all the time your well-meaning friends and relatives will eventually turn you into a complete invalid – they will change your life for you and they will allow you to be dominated completely by your arthritis.

Your friends and relatives will, of course, do these things because they love you, because they don't like to see you suffering and because they feel sympathetic towards you. But although the sympathy, attention and physical help you get because of your disease will enable you to avoid work, gardening, household chores (and even sex if you want) your life will be changing and there is a real risk that the change will be permanent.

Gradually, your friends will teach you to behave like an invalid. You will slowly but certainly move away from living a normal life. Because you do not have to make the effort to walk to the corner shop or to pick up your newspaper your joints will stiffen up and eventually you will find that you are simply not able do these things even if you want to.

In the end your friends and relatives will probably feel frustrated as you become more and more of an invalid. They will feel inadequate because, despite all their efforts, your pain and disability will get worse rather than better. It is posssible that your friends will lose patience, and they won't know what else they can do to help you. They will feel embarrassed and even faintly irritated – and then they will feel guilty. Eventually their visits will become more and more infrequent.

By then, however, it will be too late for you to escape from your role as a full-time invalid. Because you will have been treated as an invalid, and encouraged to think of yourself as an invalid, you will have become one. The longer you have been bed- or chair-bound the more difficult you will find it to break free. Your life will revolve around your pain because you will not be able to do anything else with your life apart from worry about your pain. And, to make things even worse, the weaker and more dispirited you become the more susceptible to pain you will become. In addition, you will probably be addicted to pills of various kinds.

Don't say none of this will happen to you because it can and it will if you let it. Around the world it happens to thousands, probably millions, of people every year.

## LEARN TO THINK POSITIVELY

There are, however, things that you can do to stop all this happening to you – and to stop yourself being dominated by your pain and arthritis. The key is that you must try to take a strong and aggressive attitude towards your illness.

You are the only person who can do this. Other people – the people who are closest to you and the professionals who work with you – almost certainly cannot or will not do it for you. Your friends and relatives will be driven by compassion, sympathy and love and their natural response will be to get you to give in to the pain. And the chances are that the professionals looking after you will do the same. I am not, of course, suggesting that you should fight your pain or try to ignore it. As I have explained elsewhere, that sort of attitude can be dangerous too for you may damage your joints if you try to move them when they are painful and stiff.

But when your pain is less critical you must take the initiative and try to ensure that you – not your arthritis – retain control of your life. How do you do this? Well, a good starting point is to try as hard as you can to take an active and positive role in your own treatment. Learn as much as you can about your disease, about what is causing your pain, about what makes it worse and about the ways in which you can help yourself. Reading this book is an excellent starting point, for in these pages you will find a considerable amount of information about the various types of arthritis and many practical tips on how best to cope.

Ask your doctor to explain things to you when he suggests new pills or other new forms of treatment. Try to regard your arthritis and the pain it brings as an enemy that can be controlled even if it cannot be conquered or banished completely. By doing whatever you can to control your own destiny and by making a genuine effort to take a positive and aggressive role in your own treatment you will help yourself to dominate your disease and reduce the level of your pain. You should be aware, too, that if you respond to your arthritis in a passive way there will be rewards of a different type. You need to be conscious of this so that you can keep on guard and resist the temptations that will inevitably come your way.

For example, if you stay in bed all day you will be comfortable and warm and because people can see that you are ill they will probably be supportive and sympathetic. If, on the other hand, you get out of bed and walk to the shops you may be uncomfortable and the amount of sympathy you receive will probably be less. This means that getting up and going out and doing things always takes a great deal of determination and courage. To make things easier, try to make sure that you reward yourself as much as you can. When you go out to the shops arrange to meet friends for a coffee or make an extra trip and buy yourself a treat – perhaps a book or some music.

By treating your pain aggressively and by trying to dominate your arthritis you will ensure that you stay in control of your life. It might not be easy, but in the end the benefits you will receive will be inestimable.

## HEAT

If you have ever come into the house after a hard day working in the garden or after a long walk in the countryside and sunk yourself into a bathful of warm water, then you will know just how soothing and relaxing heat can be. A shower may be an efficient and cheap way of cleaning the body, but a warm bath can do things a shower simply cannot do!

Similarly, you have probably felt the immense amount of relief that a hot-water bottle can provide to aching or sore muscles.

Although scientists have studied the subject for years, no one is certain exactly how heat gets rid of pain. There are two possible explanations.

First, it may be that heat produces nerve impulses which help to stop pain impulses getting through to the brain (in exactly the same way that rubbing a sore elbow helps to stop the pain messages getting to the brain).

Secondly, it is known that when the tissues become heated the flow of blood is increased. Some scientists argue that the increased blood flow helps to get rid of chemicals such as histamine and prostaglandins which are responsible for the production of the feeling of pain.

Of course, it doesn't really matter how heat manages to get rid of pain. The important thing is that it does.

Using heat to eradicate pain is by no means a new phenomenon. In countries all around the world medical historians have shown that doctors have for centuries used hot springs and hot soaking tubs to help patients overcome their pains. It seems that the pains associated with arthritis are especially likely to be controlled or conquered with the aid of heat.

If you want to apply heat to specific areas of your body you can try using heated towels, an electrically heated pad, a sun lamp or a good old-fashioned hot-water bottle. If you do try the latter make sure that the rubber is not perished, the stopper fits and the bottle is wrapped in a towel so that it does not burn your skin.

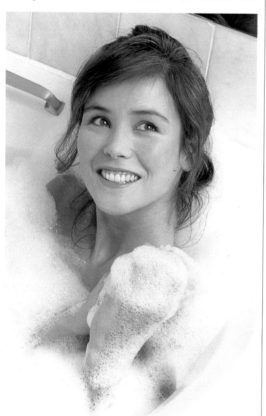

## ICE

In a recent research paper an American doctor who specializes in the treatment of pain claimed that after being massaged with ice many of his patients got relief from their pain for up to four hours at a time. The doctor reported that around three-quarters of the patients in one group had benefited by using ice.

Although the idea of using ice to treat pain may seem a rather odd one, many other doctors have experimented with it and have found that ice can sometimes be more effective than heat in the relief of pain!

How on earth can ice help to relieve pain?

One theory is that ice helps to encourage the human body to produce endorphins – special pain-relieving hormones.

Another theory is that ice stops pain messages getting through to the brain in much the same sort of way that heat does – by blocking the passage of nerve impulses to the brain.

And a third theory is that ice closes down the blood vessels and therefore makes the whole area feel numb and anaesthetized.

The ice cubes that you get out of your fridge can be used to combat pain but you have to be careful: ordinary ice cubes have sharp edges and can cut! You can get round this problem either by crushing your ice cubes and then wrapping them up in a thin cloth such as a towel or by crushing them and putting them either into a rubber bag

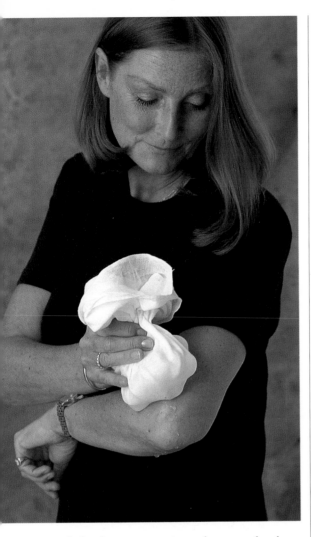

made for the purpose or into a hot-water bottle.

There is no law that says that a hot-water bottle can only be used to keep hot things hot – it can also be used to keep cold things cold!

However you wrap your ice you should rub it over the part of your body that is painful. Press fairly firmly and rub the ice either in a backwards and forwards movement or in continuous circles.

When you first start rubbing ice on your skin you should feel the cold. Then you will feel a burning and finally a little numbness and stiffness. Do take care not to hold the ice against your skin for more than five minutes at a time because ice, like heat, can burn your skin – so make sure that you keep the ice moving.

The moment that your skin starts to feel numb remove the ice and start to move the area.

## VIBRATORS

A vibrator has the same sort of effect as a TENS device, and is much more easily available.

When an ordinary vibrator was used by 17 patients suffering from facial pain and held on the relevant area for 30 minutes, 14 of the patients reported that their pain was significantly reduced both during stimulation and for some time afterwards. Eight out of the 17 patients reported that they obtained relief for between four and six hours afterwards. These patients reported that the vibrator was more effective than anything else they had tried. Most important of all, a year after the initial experiment the patients were still getting relief from their vibrators. Another research project showed that 47 out of 50 patients obtained pain relief by using a vibrator.

Ask your doctor if he or she thinks your pain could be helped in this way.

## KEEP BUSY

Many arthritis sufferers try to rest as much as they can. They are reluctant to get too involved in work or in any social activities, partly because of their pain and partly because they don't want to let other people down.

Although this is understandable it can be a mistake. Of course, it is vitally important to rest when pain is bad. But resting too much can be bad for you in the long term.

Too much inactivity can lead to muscles becoming weak and to essential organs deteriorating. And if you are inactive then the chances are high that you will become bored – and people who are bored are far more susceptible to pain than those who keep mentally active.

So, try to do as much as you comfortably can!

If your work does not provide you with the intellectual stimulation that you need, then try attending an evening class at a local college. You should find a wide variety on offer and they are usually inexpensive.

Finally, expand your personal library and your regular reading habits. A good book can help you forget your pain as well as a bottle of pills!

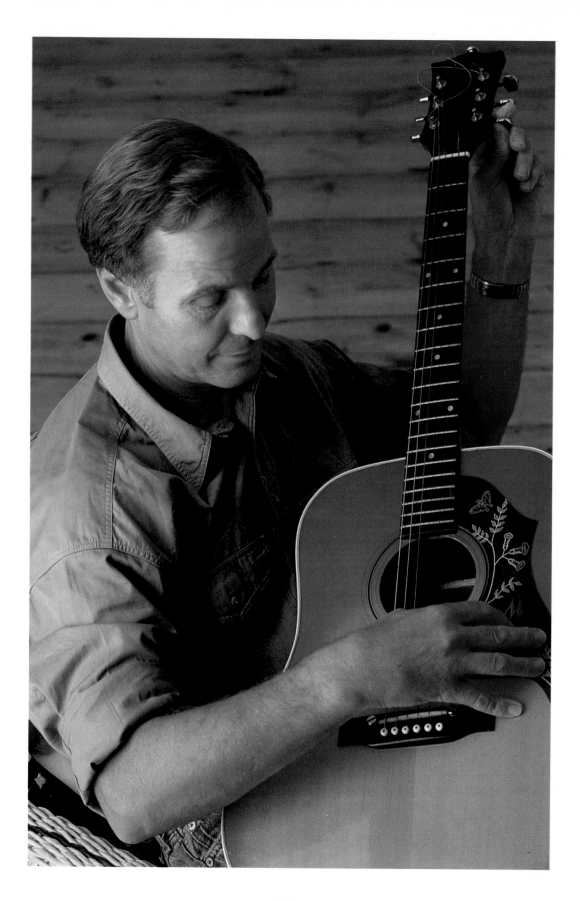

## MASSAGE

Massage is a useful way of helping to ease tension, soothe tight muscles and relieve pain (though don't let anyone massage a sore or inflamed joint – massage should never be painful).

Massage helps in several ways: it clears away the 'knots' that accumulate in your muscles when you are anxious, tense and under stress; it allows close personal contact with another person, possibly a friend, which will, in itself, provide comfort and reassurance; it stimulates the production of endorphins, the body's own pain-killing hormones; and it stimulates the production of the sensory impulses that block the transmission of pain messages to the brain. In addition, some doctors believe that massage soothes the mind.

Remember that when you automatically stretch an aching back or rub those parts of your body that ache, you are instinctively helping yourself through simple massage therapy.

## MUSIC

Many pain sufferers claim that they obtain relief by listening to music. Some say that they find classical music relaxing. Opera seems popular as a pain-reliever. And others say that rock and roll music is most effective for them. A third group enjoy special relaxation tapes – sometimes described as 'new age' music.

You can either listen to your music through ordinary speakers or through headphones. Using headphones will enable you to listen without disturbing other people. Some pain sufferers claim that they get a better result by using headphones because they can 'lose' themselves in their music more readily.

Music can be soothing and relaxing, cheering and calming.

## HOW TO SLEEP DESPITE THE PAIN

It is during sleep that we recharge our physical and mental batteries. Getting a good night's sleep is essential for all of us – and especially vital for anyone who is trying to fight a disease that is as disabling and as exhausting as arthritis.

However, if you suffer from pain caused by your arthritis then it is almost inevitable that you will have some difficulty in getting to sleep

Anyone who suffers from persistent pain will confirm that the pain seems to get worse as the day goes on, reaching its worst point fairly late in the evening – and now even the experts have confirmed that this is what happens. Anaesthetists in both Australia and Great Britain have confirmed that people who suffer from long-term pain seem to get the worst pain at around ten o'clock in the evening – just when most folk are getting ready to go to bed. Just to make things worse, anxiety, depression and other symptoms also tend to get much worse around this time too.

So, because getting a good night's sleep is so important, here are some tips that should help you if your pain keeps you awake.

**1.** If you find that pain makes sleeping at night difficult try taking a nap in the afternoon . Alternatively, try going to bed earlier in the evening before the pain gets really bad – but if you do this don't expect to be able to sleep all through the night as well. I once saw a very indignant patient who complained that he kept waking up at six o'clock every morning. When I discovered that he was going to bed at nine o'clock at night I had to explain to him that nine hours sleep was really quite enough for anyone. Another patient of mine complained that she couldn't sleep as much as she used to and then confessed that she was in the habit of taking a four-hour nap every afternoon.

**2.** Try to make sure that you don't get woken up unnecessarily once you are asleep. There are few things more annoying than having to struggle to overcome pain in order to get to sleep and then having to get out of bed an hour later to go to the lavatory. Avoid alcohol, tea, and coffee during the evening as these are stimulants and are particularly likely to keep you awake). Empty your bladder before going to bed. If you smoke then do not smoke for at least an hour or two before you go to bed and don't smoke in bed.

Make sure that you don't get woken up because you feel too cold, too hot or too uncomfortable in any other way. If your bedroom is noisy it might be worth while investing in some soundproofing (though bookshelves filled with books make an even better soundproofing system) or double glazing on your windows. Alternatively, buy and use simple ear plugs which can be very effective at keeping out noise.

**3.** Do make sure that your bed is comfortable. Many people struggle to get to sleep on a bed that is too soft or too hard. If you suffer from bad joints it is especially important that you make sure that your bed is just right for you – test a new bed before buying one. If you and your partner need beds with a different amount of spring in them you should be able to find something suitable, for beds are now made to cope with this sort of problem. By and large most people with bad joints seem to find a rather firm bed far more comfortable than one which has become soft and very saggy and has no springs left in it.

**4.** As an arthritis sufferer you will probably be especially susceptible to the cold, so make sure that you are warm! Use a warm duvet (perhaps a warmer one in winter than you use in the summer) because it will be far easier to make the bed afterwards than if you use old-fashioned sheets and blankets. And use an electric blanket or hot-water bottle to warm your bed before you get into it (though do make sure that you follow all the precautions – do not sleep in a bed when your electric blanket is switched on, do not use a hot-water bottle that is perished or has a loose-fitting stopper, make sure that your hot-water bottle is wrapped in a towel or a pillow case and never, ever use an electric blanket and a hot-water bottle at the same time).

Some arthritis sufferers find that they get relief – and go to bed physically relaxed and more supple – if they have a warm bath before retiring.

**5.** I don't think that sleeping tablets are of any real value to people who cannot sleep because of the pain of arthritis. Most sleeping tablets are now recommended only for fairly short-term use

– often for no more than two weeks or so – and although I know that millions of people do use sleeping tablets regularly I think there are dangers in doing this and very few advantages.

The main reason for my disapproval is that the most commonly prescribed sleeping tablets are in the benzodiazepine group of drugs, and these pills are capable of producing a wide range of side effects. If pills of this kind are taken for more than a fortnight or so they can start to cause sleeplessness – the very condition for which they were originally prescribed. Not realizing what is happening to him or her, the patient will probably increase the dosage and may then end up dozy, unable to think clearly and unsteady on his or her feet – but still not able to sleep properly.

It is also important to remember that most of the benzodiazepine sleeping tablets have an effect which can last much longer than one night. If you take a benzodiazepine sleeping tablet late one evening you will still be under the effects of that drug for most (if not all) of the following day. The inevitable result of this is that you will find it difficult to concentrate and so will be more likely to fall over and injure yourself. The tablet you take to help yourself get to sleep at night may well turn you into a permanent invalid.

It is also important to remember that there is evidence now available which suggests that the benzodiazepine drugs may make you more susceptible to pain! And, finally, it is also important to bear in mind that the benzodiazepine drugs can be addictive and there are currently many millions of people around the world who are hooked on these drugs. Many drug experts claim that it is harder to get off one of these drugs than it is to get off heroin. My conclusion is that the only pills you should take to help you sleep if the pain is keeping you awake should be pain-killers.

## IMAGINATION

It isn't only the real world which affects the amount of pain you feel. Your imagination can make your pain far more noticeable – and potentially far more destructive. But your imagination

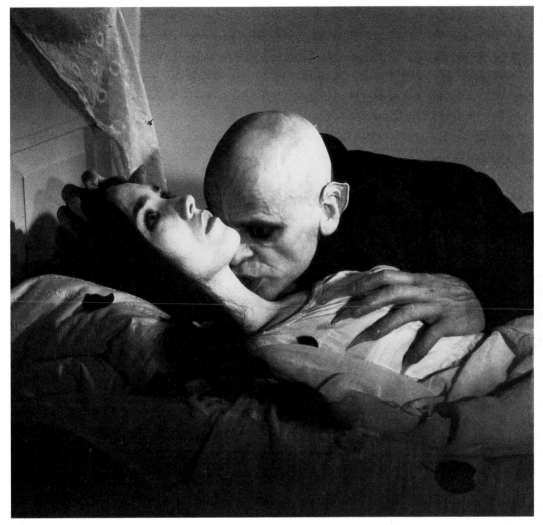

*If you watch a horror movie you'll check the doors and windows are locked before going to bed.*

can also be used to conquer your pain. The power of the imagination over the mind is well illustrated by people's reaction to films. If, for example, you are watching a scary film you will feel a sense of fear and will probably double check door and window locks even though logically you know you are in no danger – you are probably in your own sitting room with the cat on your lap.

In an experiment patients were asked to concentrate on the parts of their bodies where their pains were strongest. They were then asked to imagine that their pain had a 'shape' and had a red line drawn all around it. Next, they were told to imagine that their pain area was getting slowly smaller and smaller. Amazingly, the patients reported that as their imagined pain areas shrank so did the amount of pain they were feeling!

## Laughter

The amount of pain that you suffer will depend to a very large extent upon your moods and the frame of your mind. If you are feeling low and bored then you will be far more likely to notice your pain than if you are feeling cheerful and deeply involved in something.

It may be an exaggeration to describe laughter as the best medicine, but it is no exaggeration to describe it as one of the best ways to tackle and defeat pain. See pages 40–3 for further information about arthritis and emotion.

# CHAPTER SIX

# The Importance of Diet

*Numerous claims have been made about the importance of diet to arthritis sufferers. Some 'experts' have claimed that special food supplements will help delay the onset of arthritic symptoms. Others have argued that avoiding fruit wil help relieve symptoms such as pain and stiffness.*

## DIETING FACTORS IN ARTHRITIS

Today it seems clear that there are only two important dietary factors which influence arthritis (though there are some special dietary restrictions associated with gout – see pages 64–5).

First, you will be more likely to suffer from arthritis – and more likely to suffer from it badly – if you are overweight because your joints will be constantly under unnecessary pressure. This is particularly true of your weight-bearing joints – the hips, knees, ankles and spine. The more excess fat you carry the worse the problem will be. Losing weight, and staying slim, is essential if you are to protect your joints. There is a section on how to lose weight – and stay slim for ever – on pages 50–6 and 58–9.

Secondly, you will also reduce the risk of developing arthritis if you eat a vegetarian diet and avoid meat completely. This will also help to control and minimize your symptoms if you are already an arthritis sufferer. Recent research showed that patients with rheumatoid arthritis who followed a vegetarian diet enjoyed a significant reduction in the amount of pain they suffered, in the number of tender and swollen joints they had and in the amount of stiffness they had to endure in the morning. Blood tests also showed that the disease had been brought under better control.

You do *not* need to stop eating milk or eggs in order to benefit from this diet, though you should try to keep your consumption of dairy produce (milk, cheese and butter) to a minimum. (It is particularly important that you do not replace the meat in your diet with cheese since this can lead to an unhealthy 'high fat' diet and can also trigger a dairy produce allergy).

## HOW TO BECOME A VEGETARIAN

Cutting meat out of your diet is easier than it sounds. Most of us are brought up to regard meat as the central part of any main meal and as a result we feel slightly 'lost' and uncomfortable when we try to think of a week's menus that don't include any meat – our imaginations just can't conjure up a list of dishes and a shopping basket full of ingredients.

If you don't spend a little time preparing yourself for vegetarianism you will probably end up eating a constant diet of cheese sandwiches and cheese omelettes. If you do this two things will happen. First, you will probably make yourself ill because most cheeses contain quite a lot of fat and you could easily end up eating more fat than you were doing when you were eating meat! Secondly, you will soon become so bored that you will begin to wonder whether arthritis wouldn't be preferable.

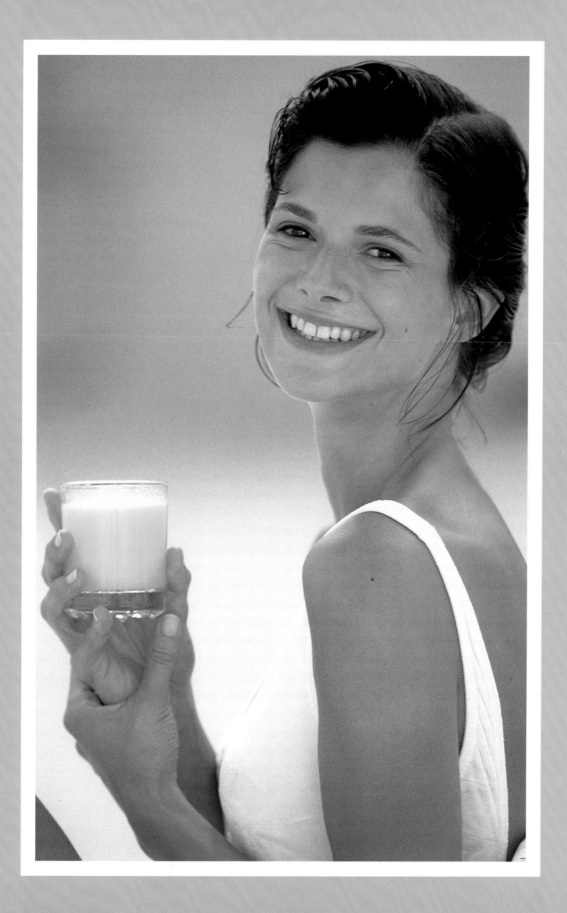

## BASIC FACTS ABOUT FOODSTUFFS

Food provides both the building blocks which enable your body to grow and to maintain and repair itself and the fuel which enables you to stay active and alive, to keep warm and to use your muscles. In order to make sure that you eat a healthy, balanced diet you must first understand a little about food – what nutrients it contains and what your body needs.

## FATS

Your body gets much of the energy it needs from the fat you eat. Some fat in your diet is essential.

However, most of us eat far too much fat – with the result that unwanted supplies are stored as 'body fat' in all the old and far too familiar places. If you eat an ordinary diet that includes meat, the chances are high that most of your fat intake will come from meat and meat products and from dairy products such as milk, butter and cream. Changing to a good vegetarian diet will almost certainly dramatically reduce your intake of fat (and will, therefore, probably help you to lose any unnecessary weight and to stay slim).

All types of fat contain the same number of calories and are made up of the same basic fatty acid building blocks: saturated fatty acids, unsaturated fatty acids and polyunsaturated fatty acids. The differences between the make-up of fatty foods depend upon the proportion of saturated to unsaturated fatty acids. You can tell whether a fatty food contains a preponderance of saturated or unsaturated fatty acids just by looking at it, for fats which contain a lot of saturated fatty acids are usually hard at room temperature (like lard and butter) whereas fats that mostly contain unsaturated or polyunsaturated fatty acids (such as most vegetable oils) are usually liquid.

It is saturated fats, which commonly come from meat and dairy products, which cause most trouble. Our bodies cannot digest saturated fats properly and so when you eat a meal that contains a lot of saturated fat the fat stays in your bloodstream, clinging to the inner lining of your blood vessels and eventually producing a narrowing that can lead to high blood pressure, heart disease and other circulatory disorders. The presence of large quantities of saturated fat in your bloodstream also stops your body metabolizing food properly and leads to the development or exacerbation of diseases as varied as gout and diabetes. Polyunsaturated fatty acids are far more essential, since they are needed for the maintenance of cell membranes and for the production of important

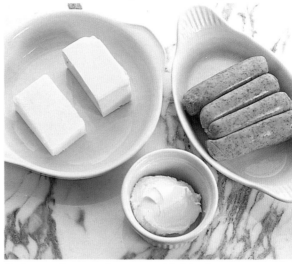

*Dairy products and meat are high in fat.*

substances such as prostaglandins which have a host of vital functions.

Whenever the subject of 'fat' arises the subject of 'cholesterol' comes up too – and I doubt if there is any aspect of food that causes more confusion. Cholesterol, which is present in all animal tissues, has some similar properties to fat but is recognized as being potentially dangerous because if the level of cholesterol in your blood reaches too high a concentration then it can increase your chances of having a heart attack.

Cholesterol is present in many ordinary foods (cheese, chocolate, cream, eggs, heart, kidneys, liver, crab, lobster, brains, caviar) but most of the cholesterol in our bodies comes not from foods that contain cholesterol but from other fatty foods. Our bodies can make their own cholesterol from saturated fats, so if your diet contains a high quantity of saturated fat your body will make more cholesterol and your blood cholesterol level will probably rise. (Unsaturated fats provide the same amount of energy as saturated fats but tend to *reduce* blood cholesterol levels).

By adopting a vegetarian diet you will automatically reduce your intake of saturated fats, and therefore help keep your body's cholesterol level down. Cutting down your total fat intake will cut down your calorie intake and help you to lose weight. It is, however, important to remember that you will only reduce your intake of saturated fatty acids if you are careful to ensure that you do not replace meat with too much dairy produce.

## PROTEINS

You need to eat a balanced supply of protein because protein is essential for growth, for the repair of damaged tissues and for the production of some vital enzymes. The protein in your body contains long chains of amino acids (of which there are 22 types) and your protein is created from the amino acids you obtain from proteins you eat. Protein is, indeed, so necessary that if your diet contains too little then tissue proteins – particularly muscles – will be broken down and cannibalized so that you can stay alive.

On the other hand, if your diet contains more protein than your body needs the constituent amino acids will be broken down and some of the protein will be turned into fat. There are other hazards in eating too much protein: it can put a strain on your kidneys and your liver (because large amounts of amino acid have to be broken down) and can increase the loss of calcium from your body (with an increased risk of osteoporosis developing). Some experts also believe that a diet that contains too much protein (that usually means one that includes a lot of meat) may lead to an increased risk of cancer and heart disease. Women who live in Japan and eat a diet that contains relatively little meat run a low risk of developing breast cancer; those living in America and eating approximately four times as much meat are far more likely to be susceptible.

Eight of the amino acids that are used to create adult proteins and 10 of the amino acids that create proteins in children have to be obtained in the food we eat because our bodies cannot make them from scratch. These amino acids are, therefore, known as 'essential' and in the past the foods (mostly meat) which were regarded as containing good supplies of the essential amino acids were

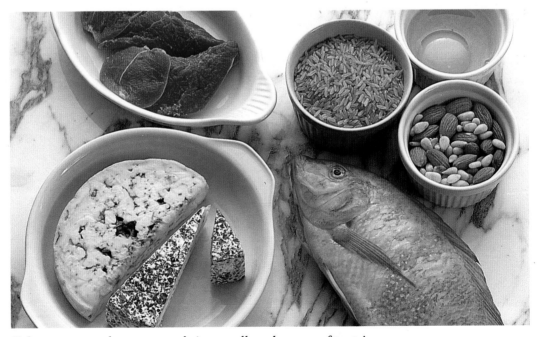

*Fish, nuts, meat, cheese, eggs and rice are all good sources of protein.*

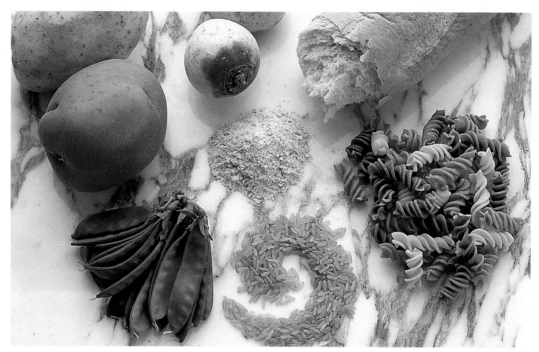

*It is now known that plant proteins can provide sufficient amino acids in your diet.*

called 'first-class proteins'. Plant proteins, which were believed not to contain adequate quantities of the 'essential' amino acids, were known as 'second-class'. This difference led to a discrimination against vegetarianism by nutritionists who regarded a non-meat diet as inadequate.

Today, however, it is recognized that any balanced diet will contain all the amino acids needed to create new body protein and you can get all the amino acids your body requires without eating any meat or meat products at all. Even vegans – who eat neither eggs nor dairy produce – can get an adequate supply of protein-building amino acids from the plants they eat. Meat is only a marginally better source of protein than nuts and seeds and is no better than soya beans. Once the proteins are inside your body they will be broken down and the various amino acids will then be used to build up the proteins your body needs. It doesn't matter where you get your proteins from.

## CARBOHYDRATES

Carbohydrates are manufactured by plants which use water, sunlight and carbon dioxide to make them. There are three basic types of carbo-

hydrate: starches (complex carbohydrates), sugars (simple carbohydrates) and fibre (or roughage).

## STARCHES

Foods such as pulses (peas and beans), cereals, rice, pasta and many different types of fruit and vegetable are rich in starches which are digested slowly when eaten. If you become a vegetarian your intake of starches will probably increase. Starches contain a considerable amount of potential energy and a wide range of other essential

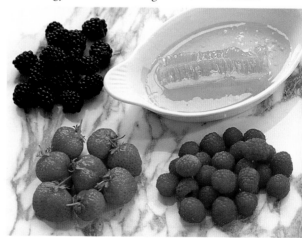

*Keep your intake of all sugars down.*

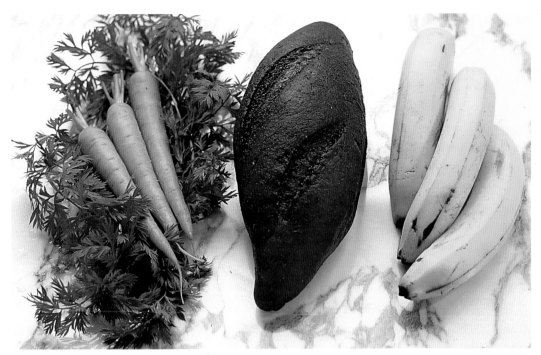

*Rye bread and most vegetables and fruits will add soluble fibre to your diet.*

nutrients including proteins, vitamins and minerals. Starchy carbohydrates are fairly low in calories.

## SUGARS

The sugars we most commonly use are the refined white or brown varieties and these types of sugar – derived from sugar cane or sugar beet – are also known as sucrose. Sucrose is rich in calories but contains very few other ingredients. However, sucrose is not the only type of sugar. Others, which include honey, treacle, corn syrup, glucose, fructose and maltose, do contain other ingredients. For example, honey contains a few vitamins and minerals. Nevertheless, these other ingredients are in fairly small quantities and there are no forms of sugar which are good for you other than as a source of 'instant' energy – and it does cause obesity and tooth decay. Despite its relative worthlessness most of us eat far too much sugar. The best way to cut down is to avoid processed foods since manufacturers add sugar to just about everything from soup (to improve the texture and flavour) to tinned meat (to keep it soft) to tomato sauce (to keep it smoother running) and to biscuits (to make them crunchy and crumbly).

## FIBRES

For years food manufacturers have been taking fibre out of our food. Now doctors know that anyone who eats a low-fibre diet will be at risk of developing all sorts of illnesses, including bowel cancer, diverticular disease of the bowel, appendicitis, gallstones and varicose veins. Fibre comes from plant cell walls and is made up of a number of complex carbohydrates. There are two main types: soluble and insoluble. The richest sources of soluble fibre are pulses (peas and beans) and products such as porridge, pearl barley or rye bread that contain oats, barley or rye. Most vegetables and fruits also contain soluble fibre. Once inside you, soluble fibre forms a sticky substance in your intestines which limits the amount of fat you absorb. It also slows down the rate at which your body absorbs sugar. Insoluble fibre is found mainly in vegetables such as spring greens and in products such as bread and breakfast cereals which are made from wheat. It acts like a sponge, swelling up as it soaks up the moisture inside us and thus making us feel full and stopping us eating more than we really need. A vegetarian diet will contain a lot of fibre.

# VITAMINS AND MINERALS

Vitamins and minerals are essential: they help to keep your body and skin healthy, they produce essential enzymes, they turn food into energy, they keep your nerves in good condition and they aid in the production of blood cells and hormones. Without vitamins and minerals you would die.

Many people who give up eating meat worry that their diet will not contain enough of these essential 'micro-nutrients' but this fear is entirely baseless since you can get all the vitamins and minerals you need from a balanced vegetarian diet. Indeed, meat-eaters are more likely to suffer from vitamin C deficiency and iron-deficiency anaemia than vegetarians are. If you eat a sensible, well-balanced diet you will not need vitamin or mineral supplements.

## VITAMIN A

Helps your body to fight infection by keeping cell walls strong. It also improves your ability to see in dim light. Carrots and green vegetables are both excellent sources of vitamin A.

## VITAMIN B1 (THIAMINE)

Helps to turn carbohydrates into energy and helps to keep heart and central nervous system healthy. Cereals, nuts, beans, eggs and peas contain B1.

## VITAMIN B2 (RIBOFLAVIN)

Helps to turn carbohydrates into energy. Eggs, milk, cheese and some green vegetables contain vitamin B2.

## VITAMIN B3 (NICOTINIC ACID OR NIACIN)

Helps to keep brain, skin and gastrointestinal tract healthy. Wholemeal cereals contain B3.

## VITAMIN B6 (PYRIDOXINE)

Plays a vital role in the way enzymes metabolize amino acids and proteins. Cereals, fruit and vegetables all contain vitamin B6.

## VITAMIN B12 (CYANCOBALAMIN)

Vital for the formation of red blood cells and plays a part in the functioning of the central nervous system. Eggs, dairy products, soya milk, yeast extracts and margarines contain it.

## VITAMIN C (ASCORBIC ACID)

Helps form connective tissue and helps to fight infections and absorb iron. Fresh fruit and fresh vegetables contain it.

## VITAMIN D (CHOLCALIFEROL)

Helps absorb and use calcium and phosphorus for the production of strong bones and teeth. Eggs and dairy produce contain it but most of us can make all the vitamin D we need from the action of sunshine on our skin.

## VITAMIN E (TOCOPHEROL)

Has an exaggerated reputation and deficiency in humans is virtually unknown. Green leafy vegetables, vegetable oils and eggs contain vitamin E.

## VITAMIN K (NAPTHOQUINONE)

Plays a vital role in blood-clotting mechanism. Fresh, green, leafy vegetables such as broccoli, cabbage, lettuce and spinach all contain it.

## IRON

Essential for the manufacture of red blood cells. Cabbage, spinach, kale, beans, peas and dried fruit all contain it.

## CALCIUM

Helps form the structure of bones and teeth. Dark green vegetables, beans, milk and cheese all contain it.

## ZINC

Essential for the proper functioning of the body's enzymes. Wholemeal breads, wholegrain cereals and dried beans contain it.

# Ten Questions About Becoming a Vegetarian

**1. QUESTION** Won't I be short of vitamins and minerals if I stop eating meat?

**ANSWER** A vegetarian diet which includes some dairy produce (milk, cheese and so on) and eggs will provide you with all the essential nutrients that your body needs.

**2. QUESTION** I thought iron was only available in meat.

**ANSWER** You don't need to eat meat to get a good intake of iron. Peas, beans, dried fruit and dark green vegetables such as cabbage, spinach and kale are among the vegetarian foods which are rich in iron. Vitamin C – present in large quantities in fruit and vegetables – will increase the ease with which iron is absorbed by a factor of five.

**3. QUESTION** Won't a vegetarian diet be short on essential proteins?

**ANSWER** Animal products are, pound for pound, only a very slightly better source of protein than nuts or seeds and no better than soya beans.

**4. QUESTION** If I stop eating meat won't I become weak and easily tired?

**ANSWER** No. Vegetarians have won medals in strength and endurance events and triathlon championships are regularly won by vegetarians.

**5. QUESTION** Apart from helping my arthritis will becoming a vegetarian have any other good effects on my health?

**ANSWER** A vegetarian diet will include less fat than a meat-based diet (unless you eat too many dairy foods). You will, therefore, be less likely to suffer from a wide range of disorders known to be associated with a high fat consumption.

**6. QUESTION** Is it safe for children to follow a vegetarian diet?

**ANSWER** If a child has a balanced vegetarian diet which contains a healthy mixture of fresh foods – including dairy produce and eggs – then he or she will get all the protein, vitamins and minerals that are needed.

**7. QUESTION** Will a vegetarian diet help me to lose weight?

**ANSWER** Yes, you should be able to lose weight more readily if you switch to a vegetarian diet because by changing your eating habits you will have a chance to get rid of all the old, bad habits that helped to make you fat.

**8. QUESTION** Will a vegetarian diet be more expensive than a meat diet?

**ANSWER** On the contrary, a vegetarian diet will probably be cheaper.

**9. QUESTION** Won't I find a vegetarian diet extremely boring?

**ANSWER** If you think of a vegetarian diet as being dull that must be because you have been brought up to think of meat as an essential centre-point to every meal. The truth is, however, that vegetables, fruits, pulses and cereals can make an attractive and exciting diet.

**10 QUESTION** Won't I find it difficult to eat out if I become a vegetarian? What will I do when I'm travelling?

**ANSWER** If you are booking an airline ticket tell the booking clerk that you are vegetarian. If you are booking a table at a restaurant make sure that they serve vegetarian food. It is getting easier and easier to eat out without eating meat.

# CHAPTER SEVEN

# Rest Or Exercise?

*As an arthritis sufferer it is vital that you know when to rest and when to exercise. Too much exercise can cause pain and damage your joints, but too little can lead to your joints becoming stiff and unusable – and can, in the long run, create more pain.*

## WHEN REST IS BEST

When your joints are inflamed they must be rested – and your whole body may need to be rested if you suffer from an inflammatory or auto-immune disorder. However, if you rest too much your joints will get stuck in one position and your muscles will waste away. It is important, therefore, that you establish a daily exercise programme which is designed to keep you as supple and strong as possible. It is much better to do a small amount of exercise every day than a large amount once a week.

## EXERCISE RULES FOR RHEUMATOID ARTHRITIS

**1.** Rest is important for sufferers of this disease. If your joints are swollen, stiff and painful then you must rest completely – ideally in bed.
**2.** Try to use affected joints for short periods of time only. It is important to try to exercise a joint during the periods when it is not painful so that you can keep it mobile and prevent it from becoming stiff and unusable.

## EXERCISE RULES FOR OSTEOARTHRITIS

**1.** General rest is not normally necessary for sufferers from osteoarthritis as this disease usually affects individual joints – but any joint which is painful should be rested.
**2.** Stiffness can set in if a joint is allowed to

'set' in the same position for more than an hour or so. You should, therefore, put all your affected joints through the full range of possible movements every hour at least. Exercise your joints before going to bed at night and again first thing in the morning.
**3.** Do not avoid exercise just because your joints ache a little or are stiff. You should never exercise when your joints are painful but you should try to exercise as much as you can when they are not painful.
**4.** If, after exercise, an affected joint aches more than usual – and the ache lasts for two hours or more – then your exercise programme is too severe for you and needs to be reviewed and downgraded.

## EXERCISE RULES FOR ANKYLOSING SPONDYLITIS

Mobility rather than rest is the key to the treatment of ankylosing spondylitis. It is important that you try to keep your joints moving even if they feel slightly stiff and sore; if you allow your joints to rest too much there is a risk that they will seize up completely. But don't exercise if it causes pain – talk to your doctor.

### IMPORTANT:
**BEFORE BEGINNING ANY EXERCISE PROGRAMME YOU SHOULD ALWAYS CONSULT YOUR OWN FAMILY DOCTOR.**

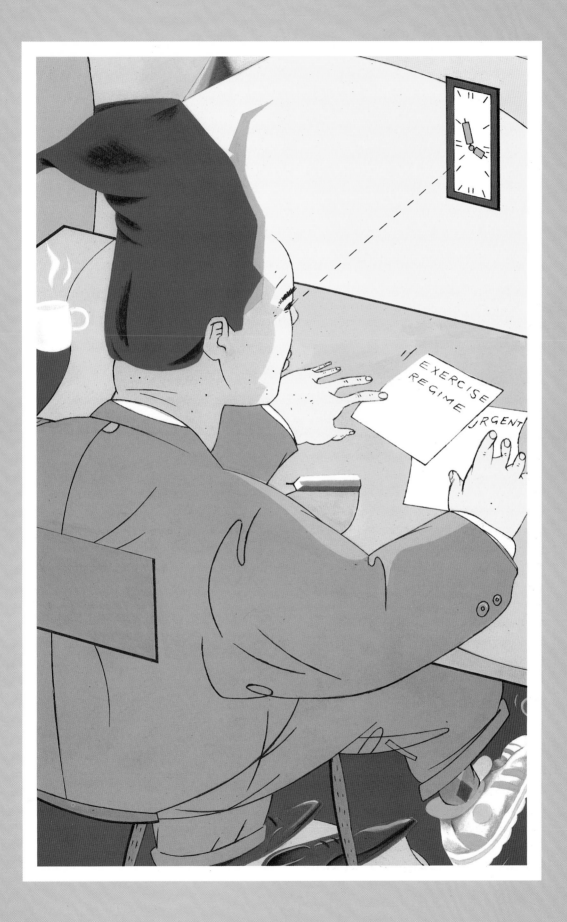

## PROTECT YOUR JOINTS WHENEVER YOU CAN

Even though you need to exercise your joints regularly – and you should carry on life as normally as possible – you must take care not to put too much of a strain on any joint in your body.

Here are some tips which are specially designed to help you protect your joints from unnecessary stresses and strains:

• **Make sure that your clothes are easy to get into and out of. Don't have buttons in inaccessible positions. Choose clothes that are roomy rather than constricting.**

• **Adjust the height of your bed and of any chairs you use regularly so that you do not have to strain your back, hips or knees when getting in or out of them.**

• **Plan your day so that you don't have to go up and down stairs unnecessarily.**

• **Never wear shoes that are painful or that do not provide you with sufficient support. Avoid high-heeled shoes and make sure that your shoes are big enough. Try to wear shoes that are lightweight rather than heavy boots.**

• **Use a shoulder bag rather than a bag that you have to carry in your hand, but don't overfill it with heavy items and do switch it from shoulder to shoulder.**

• **If you have to do a lot of physical work allow yourself time to take regular breaks.**

• **Try to avoid performing any physical activities which mean putting repeated stress on one particular joint.**

• **Do not be shy about employing aids and appliances to reduce the strain on your joints (see pages 120–4).**

• **Learn how to lift properly in order to reduce the strain on your back, hips and knees.**

• **Protect the small joints in your hands by using two hands instead of one whenever possible. Use the palm of your hand and the muscles in your forearm when you need to do any heavy work - rather than putting all the strain on your fingers (for example, when turning a stiff tap or taking the top off a jar).**

## HOW TO LIFT WITHOUT PUTTING A STRAIN ON YOUR JOINTS

1. ANY LOAD CAN DAMAGE YOUR JOINTS IF YOU LIFT INCORRECTLY. ALWAYS LIFT CAREFULLY.

2. IF THERE IS A MECHANICAL HOIST OR TROLLEY AVAILABLE, USE IT. UNLOAD CUPBOARDS AND TAKE HEAVY FURNITURE APART IF POSSIBLE. IF THERE IS NOTHING ON THE OBJECT TO HOLD ON TO PUT A STRONG ROPE UNDERNEATH IT.

3. IF YOU USE A TROLLEY REMEMBER THAT PULLING USUALLY PUTS LESS STRAIN ON YOUR BODY THAN PUSHING.

4. WEAR FLAT SHOES WITH NON-SLIP SOLES AND GLOVES THAT PROVIDE A GOOD GRIP. DON'T TRY LIFTING IN UNUSUALLY LOOSE OR TIGHT CLOTHING.

5. STAND CLOSE TO THE OBJECT YOU WANT TO LIFT WITH YOUR FEET APART TO IMPROVE BALANCE. PUT ONE FOOT SLIGHTLY AHEAD.

6. BEND YOUR HIPS AND KNEES AND KEEP YOUR BACK STRAIGHT. PICK UP THE OBJECT WITH THE WHOLE OF YOUR HAND, KEEPING YOUR ARMS CLOSE IN TO YOUR BODY.

7. BRACE YOUR ABDOMINAL MUSCLES AND THEN LIFT BY STRAIGHTENING YOUR KNEES. IF THE OBJECT IS VERY HEAVY LIFT ONE END FIRST. IF YOU HAVE TO TURN, MOVE YOUR FEET AND DO NOT TWIST YOUR BODY WHILE LIFTING.

8. LIFT SMOOTHLY AND KEEP THE OBJECT CLOSE TO YOUR BODY ALL THE TIME YOU ARE HOLDING IT.

9. IF THE OBJECT IS TOO HEAVY FOR YOU PUT IT DOWN STRAIGHT AWAY.

10. WHEN PUTTING A LOAD DOWN, LOWER YOURSELF BY BENDING YOUR KNEES AND SQUATTING.

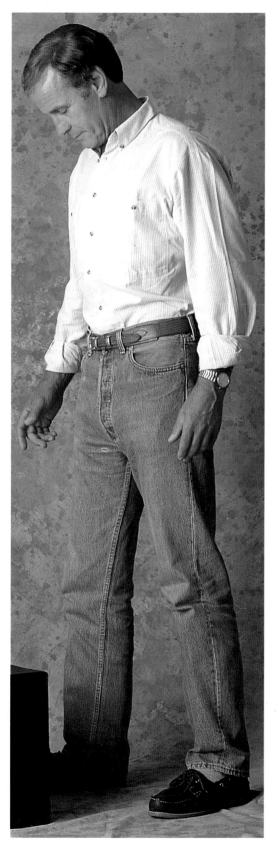

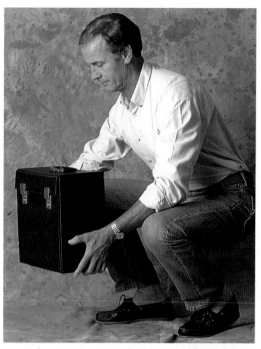

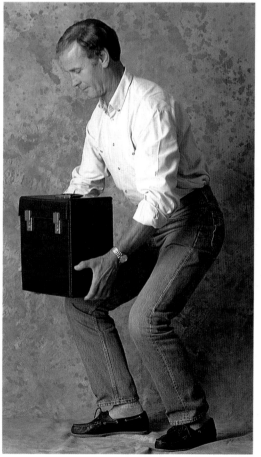

*Bend the knees rather than back when lifting.*

# Your Daily Loosening-Up Exercises

Every morning and evening you should perform the following simple exercises to get rid of as much unnecessary stiffness as you can. (Do not do any of these exercises if they cause pain.)

1. Lift up your right arm as high as you can. Keep it straight and move it around in as large a circle as you can. Now move it back in the opposite direction.

2. Hold your right arm out in front of you, bend your elbow and try to touch your right shoulder with your right hand.

3. Rotate your right hand.

4. Waggle your right hand up and down then from side to side at the wrist.

5. Exercise all the fingers of your right hand, bending and extending them individually then all together.

6. Repeat all these exercises with your left arm and hand.

7. Move your head forwards until your chin nearly touches your chest. Then move your head backwards as far as it will go.

8. Tilt your head to the right and try to touch your right shoulder with your right ear.

9. Repeat, tilting to the left instead.

10. Roll your head round gently as fully as it will go.

11. Stand up straight, bend your trunk to the right and reach down with your right hand. Try to touch the outside of your right knee with your right hand.

12. Repeat, bending to the left instead.

13. Move your hips around in as wide a circle as you can – clockwise first and then anti-clockwise.

14. Stand upright and bend your knees as far as you comfortably can.

15. Stand upright, holding on to something solid with your left hand. Move your right leg around in as large a circle as you can.

16. Stand upright, holding on to something solid with your left hand. Hold your right leg out in front of you. Now move your right foot in every possible direction.

17. Stand upright, holding on to something solid with your right hand. Move your left leg around in as large a circle as you can.

18. Stand upright, holding on to something solid with your right hand. Hold your left leg out in front of you. Now move your left foot in every possible direction.

19. Stand upright and lift yourself up until you are standing on your toes. Hold that position for as long as you can.

20. Walk around the room, taking large strides. Then walk around in the opposite direction, taking very small steps.

# EXERCISES FOR SPECIFIC JOINTS

These are useful exercises to do if you have arthritis in a particular joint.
Remember that you should try to do these exercises as often as possible in order
to keep the joint fit, supple and healthy, but you should *not* exercise when a joint is
painful and you should stop an exercise immediately if it hurts. These exercises are
also a useful way to prevent stiffness developing in an otherwise healthy joint. You
should repeat each exercise as often as you comfortably can.

## EXERCISES FOR YOUR WRISTS AND HANDS

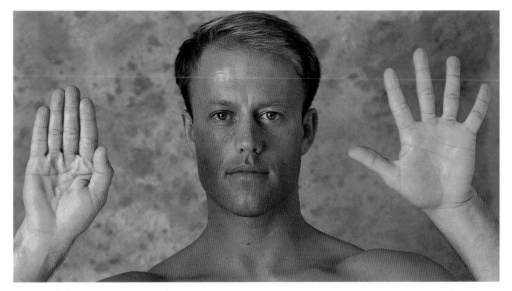

**1. SPREAD OUT YOUR FINGERS AS FAR AS YOU CAN, THEN BRING THEM IN CLOSE TOGETHER.**

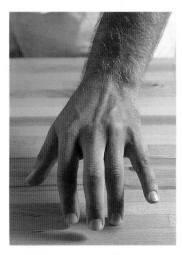

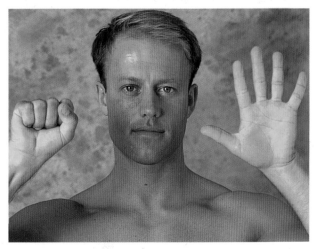

**2. REST YOUR HAND ON YOUR FINGERTIPS ON A TABLE. THEN TRY 'WALKING' YOUR HAND**

**3. FIRST MAKE A FIST, THEN STRAIGHTEN YOUR FINGERS OUT AS FAR AS YOU CAN.**

# EXERCISES FOR YOUR WRISTS AND HANDS

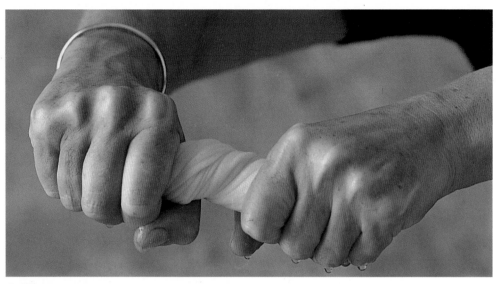

*4. Wet a cloth and try to wring it dry.*

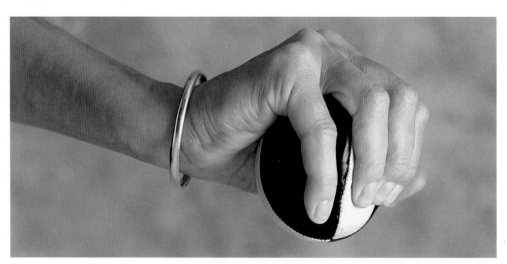

*5. Try to squeeze a rubber ball.*

*6. Make a waving movement with your hand, moving it up and down while keeping your wrist stable.*

*7. Take your thumb across to the base of your little finger.*

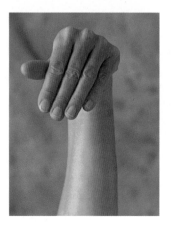

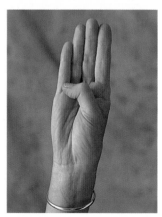

# EXERCISES FOR YOUR ELBOWS

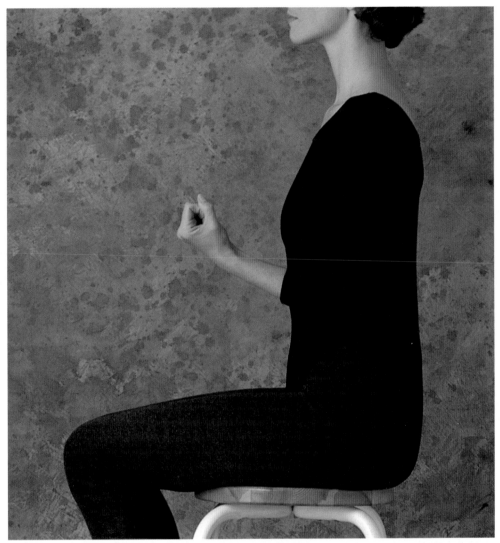

*1. SIT AS COMFORTABLY AS YOU CAN AND TRY BENDING AND STRAIGHTENING YOUR ARM AS FAR AS YOU CAN.*

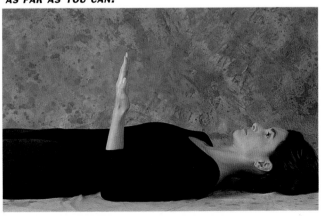

*2. LIE ON YOUR BACK WITH YOUR ARMS BY YOUR SIDE, PALMS DOWN. THEN BEND YOUR ELBOW AND TURN YOUR PALM INWARDS. NEXT, BRING IT AS CLOSE TO YOUR SHOULDER AS YOU CAN. TAKE THE HAND BACK. REPEAT THE EXERCISE WITH THE OTHER ARM.*

# EXERCISES FOR YOUR SHOULDERS

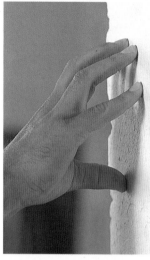

**1.** *STAND FACING A WALL. PLACE ONE HAND FLAT ON THE WALL AND BY CONTRACTING AND EXPANDING YOUR FINGERS MAKE YOUR HAND CRAWL UP THE WALL AS FAR AS IT WILL GO. SEE HOW FAR YOU ARE ABLE TO GO, THEN TRY THE EXERCISE AGAIN LATER. IF YOU DO THIS EXERCISE DAILY YOU WILL BE ABLE TO MEASURE YOUR PROGRESS.*

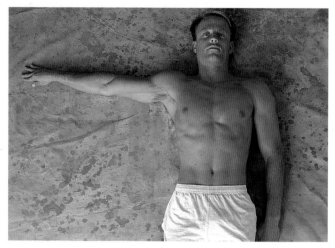

**2.** *LIE FLAT ON THE FLOOR WITH YOUR ARMS BY YOUR SIDES. MOVE YOUR RIGHT ARM AWAY FROM YOUR BODY, AS FAR AS IT WILL GO, THEN BRING IT BACK. REPEAT THIS EXERCISE SEVERAL TIMES THEN DO THE SAME WITH YOUR LEFT ARM.*

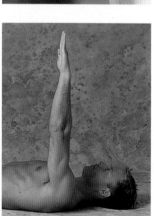

**3.** *LIE FLAT ON THE FLOOR. RAISE YOUR ARM SLOWLY UNTIL IT IS VERTICAL, THEN LOWER IT SLOWLY.*

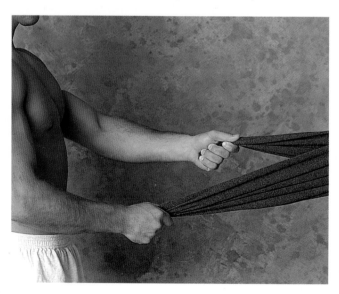

**4.** *LOOP A SCARF AROUND SOMETHING SOLID – A TABLE LEG OR DOOR HANDLE FOR EXAMPLE – AND HOLD ONE END IN EACH HAND. PULL ONE END SO THAT YOUR OTHER ARM IS PULLED IN AND THEN ALTERNATE.*

# EXERCISES FOR THE JOINTS IN YOUR NECK

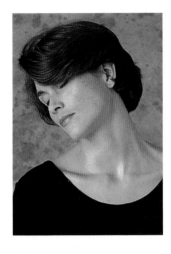 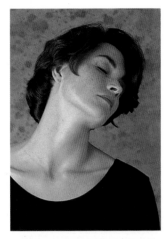

**1.** *MOVE YOUR HEAD ROUND AND ROUND, FIRST IN A CLOCKWISE DIRECTION AND THEN ANTI-CLOCKWISE.*

**2.** *MOVE YOUR HEAD TO THE RIGHT SO THAT YOU GET YOUR RIGHT EAR AS CLOSE TO YOUR RIGHT SHOULDER AS YOU CAN AND THEN REPEAT TO THE LEFT SO THAT YOU GET YOUR LEFT EAR AS CLOSE TO YOUR LEFT SHOULDER AS YOU CAN.*

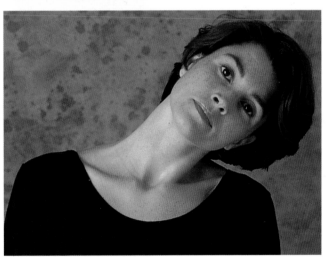

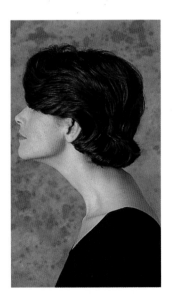 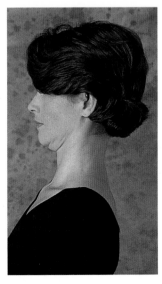

**3.** *MOVE YOUR HEAD AS FAR FORWARDS AS YOU CAN AND THEN AS FAR BACKWARDS AS YOU CAN.*

# Exercises for the Joints in Your Spine

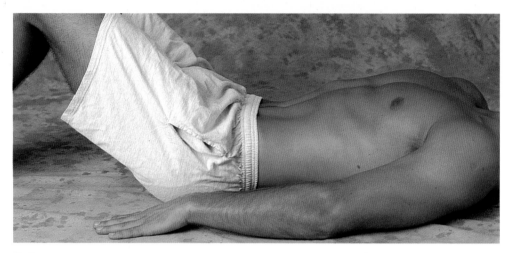

*1. Lie on your back, bend your knees, then pull in your tummy muscles.*

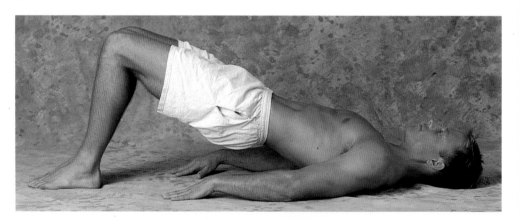

*2. Lie on your back and lift your bottom off the floor.*

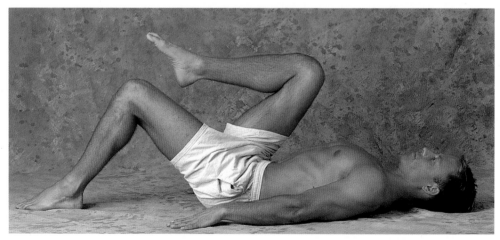

*3. Lie on your back with your knees bent and your feet on the floor, then raise your right knee up towards your chest. Repeat the exercise with your left knee.*

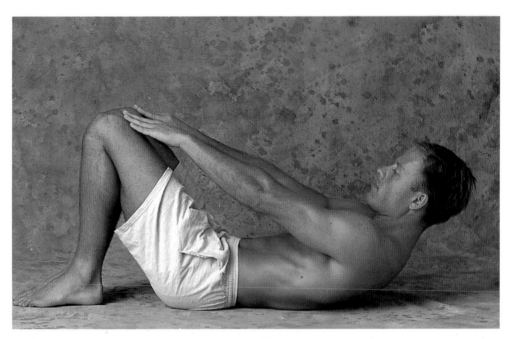

**5.** *Lie on your back with your knees bent. Try to sit up and touch your knees.*

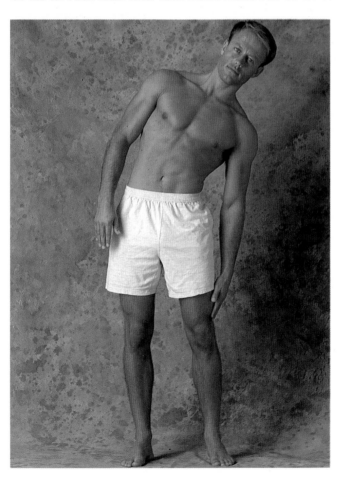

**6.** *Stand with your feet apart, your knees slightly bent, and bend sideways. Try to touch the outside of your right knee with your right hand. Then try to touch the outside of your left knee with your left hand.*

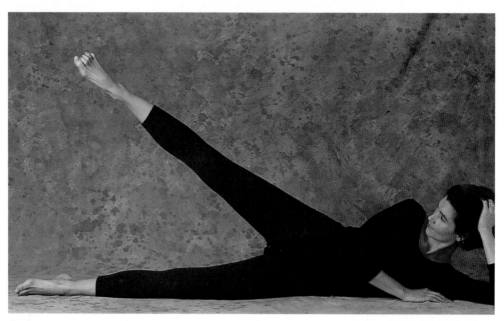

**1.** *Lie on your side on a fairly firm surface. Lift your uppermost leg straight up, away from the lower leg.*

**2.** *Lie on your back with your legs apart. Slowly move your left leg as far away from your right leg as you can. Repeat the exercise with the other leg.*

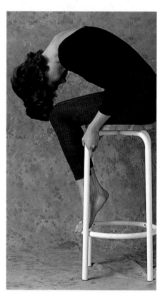

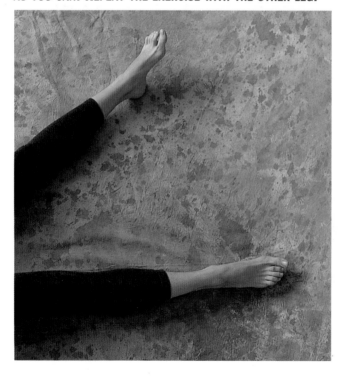

**3.** *Sit on a stool or an upright chair. Try to put your head as near to your knees as possible.*

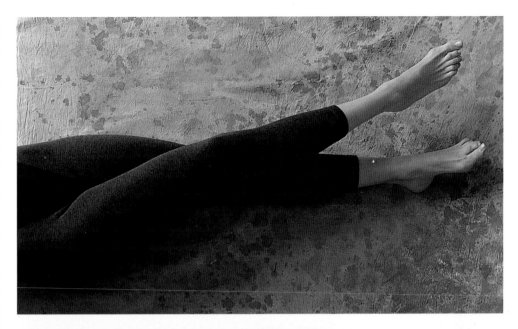

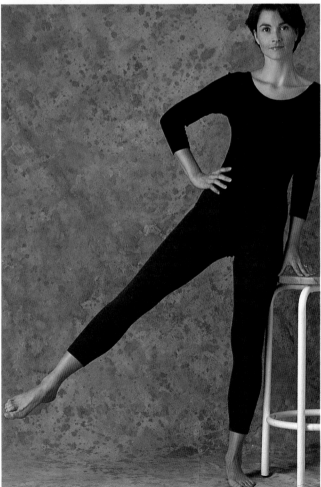

**4.** *Lie flat on your back on the floor or on a bed and try crossing one leg over the other. Then repeat the exercise with the other leg.*

**5.** *Stand upright and hold on to a stool or the back of a chair. Keep one leg straight and move the other leg round and round.*

# EXERCISES FOR YOUR KNEES

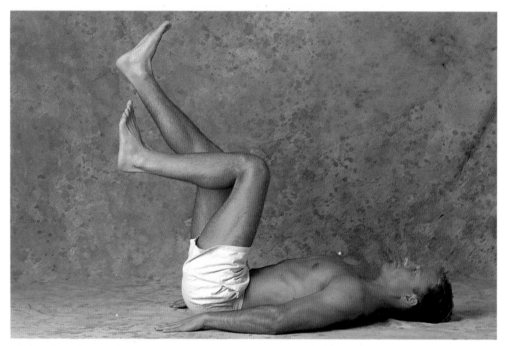

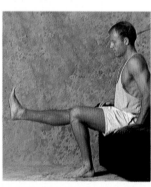

1. LIE FLAT ON YOUR BACK, LIFT YOUR LEGS IN THE AIR AND PEDAL AN IMAGINARY BICYCLE.

2. SIT ON THE EDGE OF A BED WITH YOUR LEGS HANGING DOWN, THEN STRAIGHTEN ONE LEG. LIFT THE LEG AS HIGH AS YOU CAN. REPEAT THE EXERCISE WITH THE OTHER LEG.

3. LIE ON YOUR BACK, BEND ONE LEG AS MUCH AS YOU CAN AND THEN STRAIGHTEN IT AGAIN. GET YOUR HEEL AS CLOSE TO YOUR BOTTOM AS YOU CAN.

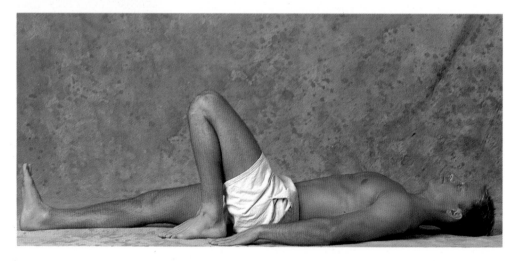

# EXERCISES FOR YOUR FEET AND ANKLES

**1.** *SIT WITH YOUR FEET FLAT ON THE FLOOR. THEN RAISE YOUR HEELS AS HIGH AS YOU CAN.*

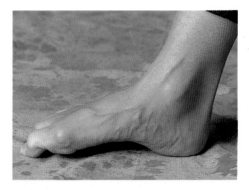

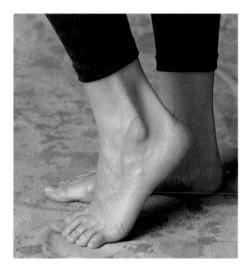

**2.** *SIT WITH YOUR FEET FLAT ON THE FLOOR. KEEP YOUR TOE AND HEEL ON THE GROUND AND LIFT THE CENTRE OF YOUR FOOT.*

**3.** *SIT WITH YOUR LEGS CROSSED AND BEND THE FOOT THAT IS IN THE AIR AS FAR AS POSSIBLE. REPEAT WITH OTHER FOOT.*

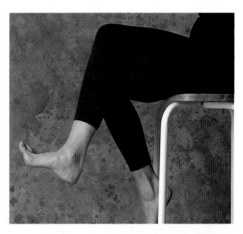

**4.** *SIT WITH YOUR LEGS CROSSED. CIRCLE YOUR FOOT ROUND AND ROUND, DRAWING A LARGE IMAGINARY CIRCLE IN THE AIR WITH YOUR BIG TOE. REPEAT WITH OTHER FOOT.*

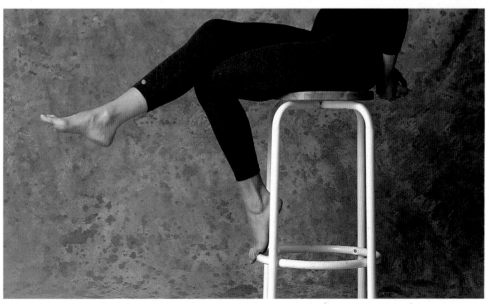

## THE IMPORTANCE OF GENERAL EXERCISE

A good general exercise programme won't stop you getting back pains but it certainly could help strengthen your general level of fitness, increase your resistance to muscular stresses and strains and reduce your susceptibility to backache and to joint problems.

If you are unfit, taking up exercise could be dangerous; if you suddenly throw yourself into a hectic exercise programme you could seriously injure yourself. However, not doing any exercise is even worse.

Most of us live fairly sedentary lives. We travel in motor cars, buses and trains and we use gadgets and machines to help us cut down the workload in the house and garden. If you doubt me, just count the number of hours you spend sitting down each day.

But your body needs exercise. In a few thousand years' time we may well have adapted to our sedentary existence, but at the moment your body is still designed for action.

Many of the diseases which are commonest today are partially caused by the fact that the majority of us simply do not exercise enough. Below is a list of just some of the diseases that can be made worse by not doing any exercise and made better by following a well-thought-out general exercise programme:

**BACKACHE:** sitting or standing in one position for long periods can result in strains that can cause long-term back trouble. A good, regular exercise programme will help to maintain your back in good condition and help to prevent future problems developing.

**ARTHRITIS:** your joints need to keep moving or else they'll seize up.

**HEADACHES:** without exercise tension builds up in your muscles and pains in the head and neck develop.

**ANXIETY:** exercise is one of the best ways of getting rid of stress and tension that will otherwise build up.

**CIRCULATION PROBLEMS:** without exercise the blood will stagnate in your veins and you are more likely to suffer from cold hands, cold feet and varicose veins.

**DEPRESSION:** regular exercise can help you avoid or fight depression.

**HEART TROUBLE:** without exercise your heart will become weak and flabby – and the slightest exertion will put it under strain. A well-thought-out exercise programme will improve the power and strength of your heart.

**DIGESTIVE UPSETS:** indigestion, irritable bowel syndrome and many other digestive problems are caused by sitting around too much.

**OBESITY:** your weight is a result of the amount of food you eat and the amount you burn up through exercise; the more exercise you do the more food you'll burn up – and the slimmer you'll get. More important still, if you exercise regularly your muscle tone will improve and you'll look slimmer and healthier.

**SLEEPLESSNESS:** regular exercise will help you sleep better without pills.

So, how much and what kind of exercise should you do? The first thing you must do is check with your doctor if you are in any doubt about your fitness.

And don't just rush down to your gym and start lifting the heaviest weights you can find. Try to find a gym with a good coach, a well-run aerobics class or a sports club that you can join. A good coach will show you how to take your pulse before and after every exercise session. Within just a few weeks you should notice that your pulse will go back to its normal rate quicker and quicker after exercising. You should also notice that your normal pulse rate gets lower as you get fitter.

One of the by-products of taking up exercise is that you'll meet new friends with whom you can share the trials and tribulations of getting fit. You'll do better and get more out of your exercise programme if it is fun, so try to choose a type of exercise that you think you'll enjoy.

If you decide to exercise only when you've got a free moment you'll never do anything – you need to set aside time for a properly organized exercise programme. However, it need not be much – three sessions a week will be plenty. You should allow a full hour for each session, though to start with you probably won't be able to manage that much. If you are really pushed for time you can squeeze a useful exercise programme into just three 20-minute sessions a week.

Try to make your exercise time inviolable and give it priority over other, less vital tasks.

You don't need a lot of money to take up exercise but do buy the right gear – the best you can afford. Remember: you're not trying to look fashionable but you do need shoes that give good support and since you'll be sweating a lot when you start exercising properly you'll need clothes that can be washed often, quickly and easily.

Finally, remember the most important rule for exercise: it should never hurt. Pain is your body's way of saying stop. If you ignore a pain you will almost certainly injure yourself. Too many people think that if they hurt, then they must be doing themselves some good!

## WARNING

**1. DO NOT START AN EXERCISE PROGRAMME UNTIL YOU HAVE CHECKED WITH YOUR DOCTOR THAT THE PROGRAMME IS SUITABLE FOR YOU. MAKE SURE THAT YOU TELL HIM OR HER ABOUT ANY TREATMENT YOU ARE ALREADY RECEIVING AND ABOUT ANY SYMPTOMS FROM WHICH YOU SUFFER.**

**2. YOU MUST STOP EXERCISING IF YOU FEEL FAINT, DIZZY, BREATHLESS OR NAUSEATED OR IF YOU NOTICE ANY PAIN OR IF YOU FEEL UNWELL IN ANY WAY. GET EXPERT HELP IMMEDIATELY AND DO NOT START EXERCISING AGAIN UNTIL YOU HAVE BEEN GIVEN THE 'ALL CLEAR' BY YOUR DOCTOR.**

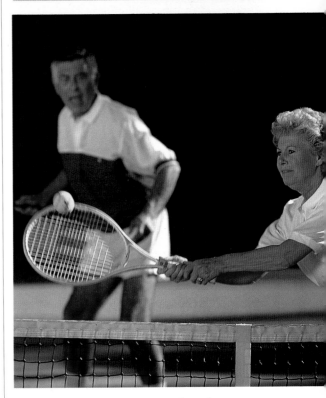

*Our bodies are not designed to be sedentary – they benefit from regular exercise.*

## WARNING: THE WRONG SORT OF EXERCISE CAN DAMAGE YOUR JOINTS

Your joints can be put under a tremendous amount of strain by any repetitive exercise. As a result arthritis – particularly osteoarthritis, in which the joints are 'worn out' – and backache are common problems among sportsmen and athletes who do not take care. Warming up beforehand, resting or even stopping when you feel tired and cooling down gently after an exercise programme are all important.

Running is one of the sports most commonly associated with back, hip and knee injuries. Running tends to tighten the lower muscles of the back, causing low back pain and increasing the risk of conditions such as ruptured disc or spondylolysis, and runners who exercise for too long on hard surfaces such as roads are particularly likely to suffer from backache. Every one hour's running means that your joints get 10,000 vibrations they don't want. Running on cambered roads means that the strains on the back are particularly bad because one leg is always running lower than the other.

But running is not, of course, the only sport that can cause joint problems. Virtually any sport can cause trouble. Over-enthusiastic swinging of a golf club, for example, can cause nasty strains that may take a long time to heal.

The most severe and potentially serious joint injuries tend to occur in contact sports such as rugby and football where a sudden jolt can cause severe damage to almost any joint.

## SWIMMING IS GOOD FOR YOU

Swimming will provide your body with an almost perfect exercise programme, improving the efficiency of your heart, muscle strength and general flexibility. It is one of the very few types of exercise that helps in these three important different ways.

Swimming will be particularly good for you if you have back or joint trouble because it will enable you to exercise without putting any stress or strain on your joints. The water will support the weight of your body and so you can exercise with the minimum of risk.

The most effective strokes are the front and back crawl which will give your whole body a good general work-out. If you swim breast stroke wear goggles and try to learn to swim without keeping your head out of the water all the time as this can put a strain on your neck.

## WALK YOUR WAY TO HEALTH

You don't have to get hot and sweaty to improve your fitness or to help strengthen your back. A gentle walk can help!

A study of golfers showed that just walking round a golf course three times a week is enough to reduce the amount of cholesterol in the bloodstream and to help get rid of excess weight! The more you enjoy your game – and the better you are able to forget your worries and anxieties – the more you will gain from it.

To benefit most from your exercise walk as briskly as you can. According to the medical journal the *Lancet*, brisk walking protects your heart just as well as more energetic exercise such as jogging or playing tennis.

## JOIN A GYM!

It is perfectly possible to get all the exercise you need for physical and mental health without ever going anywhere near a gym. But if there is a local gym I suggest that you join it! You'll benefit in several ways.

**1. It is bound to have a wider range of equipment than you can buy for yourself.**
**2. Good gyms are staffed with well-qualified instructors who can help you develop an exercise programme to suit your own needs.**
**3. You'll find that most gyms are friendly places. You will benefit enormously from the support and companionship of those around you. It is much more fun to exercise in a group than it is to exercise alone.**

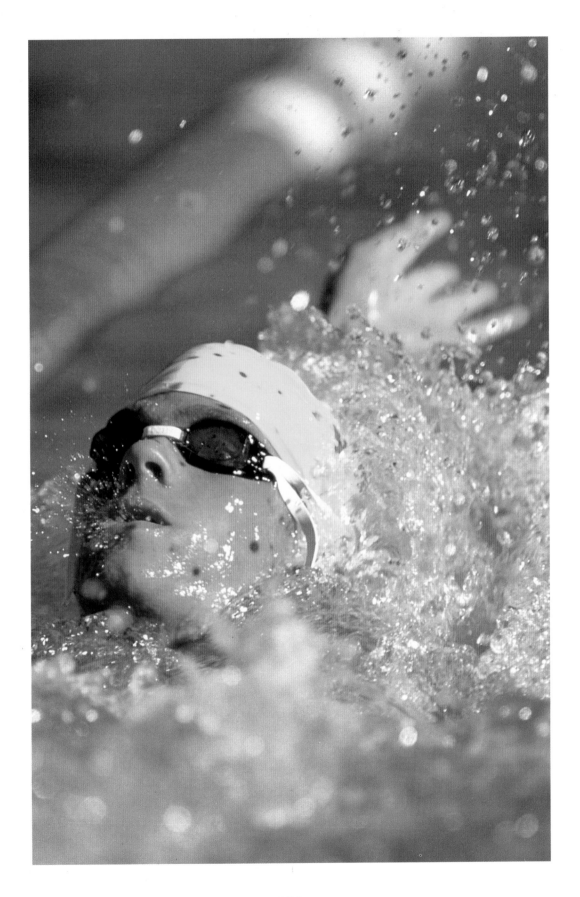

# CHAPTER EIGHT

# Alternative Solutions

*The popularity of alternative or complementary medicine has increased dramatically during the last few years. However, patients wanting to try an alternative form of healing often have difficulty in getting answers to a few basic questions such as: 'What sort of alternative medicine should I try?' 'Is it dangerous?' and 'Where do I find a good practitioner?'*

## BASIC ADVICE ABOUT ALTERNATIVE MEDICINE

Here are some simple, introductory guidelines designed to help make sure that you get the best and most appropriate alternative treatment.

**1.** Orthodox, old-fashioned doctors are, I feel, still best at dealing with emergencies. (And the great majority of the alternative specialists I have spoken to agree with this). Doctors have access to diagnostic equipment (such as X-ray machines) and to treatment facilities which are particularly useful when dealing with a patient who has an acute and life-threatening problem.

**2.** Alternative or complementary practitioners seem to be at their best when dealing with chronic or long-term problems – and arthritis is one of the diseases they seem best able to help overcome.

**3.** In many countries there are still very few regulations governing who can or cannot become an alternative practitioner. In Britain, for example, it is perfectly possible for someone with no qualifications at all to put up a plate announcing that he or she is a qualified acupuncturist, herbalist, hypnotherapist and chiropractor! There are no laws or regulations against this happening. Obviously, because this does happen it often leads to serious problems, and those

practitioners who set up in business without being properly trained have done a considerable amount of damage to the image of alternative or complementary medicine. To make sure that you visit someone who is reliable, I suggest that you ask around your friends first to see if they know of anyone whom they can recommend. Or ask your own doctor. Most doctors these days know of (and approve of) alternative medicine practitioners. And it is a myth that your doctor is likely to be cross with you if you tell him that you are planning to visit a complementary practitioner. It is not, I am afraid, safe to rely on the fact that a practitioner you are intending to visit has a list of qualifications after his name. Some of these apparently impressive qualifications can be 'bought' with very little academic effort. (My cat was once the proud owner of a huge sheaf of diplomas and paper qualifications in alternative medicine).

**4.** It is important to make sure that you visit a well-qualified and well-trained practitioner because, contrary to common belief, it is possible for alternative medicines to do harm. Patients who have visited acupuncturists using dirty needles have contracted all sorts of very nasty (and potentially lethal) disorders. Patients who

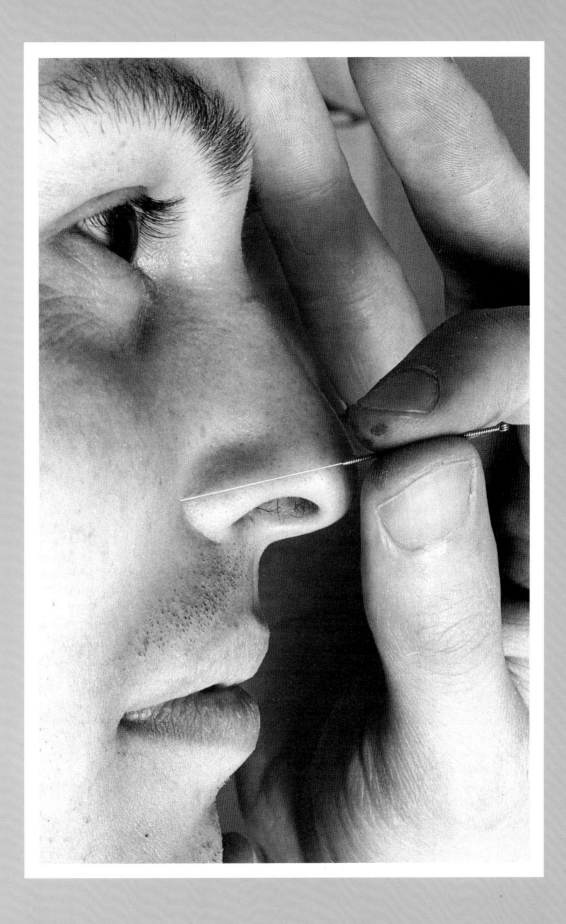

have been given contaminated herbal medicines have been made very ill. There are, I am afraid, risks with alternative medicine just as much as there are risks with orthodox medicine.

**5.** The best alternative practitioners usually practise from good, clean, well-equipped premises. Many good alternative practitioners these days practise in small groups. Personally, I would be wary of anyone who claims to be an expert in a whole range of alternative therapies. Since the training periods for subjects like acupuncture tend to be long and arduous, the very best practitioners probably specialize.

## ACUPUNCTURE

Although acupuncture was first made popular in Europe by a Dutch physician called Willem ten Rhyne, it has been used in China for over 4,000 years. Rhyne introduced acupuncture to Holland in 1683, but since then it has been regularly rediscovered by traditional Western doctors.

Some countries, such as France, have recognized the importance of acupuncture and have special acupuncture departments in many of their major hospitals.

In other countries, such as Britain, acupuncture is regarded by many traditional doctors as a 'quack remedy' that should not be taken seriously. In Britain anyone can put up a plate and claim that they are an acupuncturist. In other countries such a lax attitude to acupuncture is regarded as almost blasphemous.

Acupuncture is based upon a theory which says that the human body contains twelve meridians or channels and that it is along these channels that vital internal energies flow. However, when these meridians are blocked in some way, the flow of energy will be impeded. And it is this slowing or stopping of the flow of energy that causes illness or pain.

Acupuncturists believe that there are a number of quite specific points on the human body which can be regarded as entry points to this internal energy force. By the 14th century, Chinese doctors had identified 657 acupuncture points. Since then many other experts have been busy and today experts recognize over 1,000 acupuncture points.

The acupuncturist uses slender needles to clear the blocked meridians and release the flow of energy. The needles can be made of a variety of metals such as silver, gold or copper.

Before starting treatment the acupuncturist makes a diagnosis about the likely cause of the pain (the traditional acupuncture methods of diagnosis involve talking and listening to the patient and then identifying no less than 12 different pulses).

Once the accupuncturist has made a diagnosis he inserts his needles and manipulates them one by one. He can use several different techniques at once for manipulating the needles.

**1.** He can insert the needle and twist it backwards and forwards rather vigorously for a few seconds.

**2.** He can put one or more needles into the skin and leave it or them in place for 20 or 30 minutes.

**3.** He can connect the acupuncture needles to an electrical apparatus which passes a mild electric current through them.

**4.** He can dry and shred leaves of the Chinese wormwood plant and then burn these shredded leaves directly over an acupuncture point (this technique is known as moxibustion).

**5.** He can search out tender trigger points and insert his needles directly into those specific areas.

Despite the scepticism of the traditional medical profession there is no longer any real doubt that this technique does work. Many research papers have been published detailing the value and effectiveness of acupuncture. For example, around 20 years ago, four American surgeons reported that they had used acupuncture to treat over 300 patients in and around the New York area. The surgeons stated that in over three-quarters of the cases they had found that acupuncture is one of the most effective treatments available for skeletomuscular disorders, such as arthritis. Two doctors writing in the *Canadian Anaesthetists Society Journal* in the same year recorded that 'a large number of surgical cases operated on under acupuncture anaesthesia, with a success rate of up to 90 per cent, have now been sufficiently substantiated that the effectiveness of acupuncture can no longer be doubted'.

There is no doubt in my mind that if acupuncture had been a new 'drug' being sold by one of the world's largest and most powerful drug companies, it would have been quickly adopted by the world's traditional medical profession.

Sadly, however, acupuncture has still not found favour with most traditional doctors, some of whom regard it with suspicion because it is not something they were taught about when they were medical students. There is, I'm afraid, a powerful lobby in the medical profession which fights against 'alternative' remedies, regarding them as a professional threat. Many doctors probably fear that if they acknowledge the effectiveness of acupuncture as a remedy they may lose patients – and fees – to professional acupuncturists.

Back in 1979, acupuncture had been so widely and thoroughly tested that at a meeting of medical representatives from all six of the World Health Organization's regions it was concluded that 'the sheer weight of evidence demands that it must be taken seriously as a clinical procedure of considerable value'.

Today, the consensus seems to be that acupuncture is probably a powerful and effective way of dealing with at least 70 per cent of all long-term cases of pain. And, as I have already pointed out, acupuncture is believed to be particularly effective in the treatment of arthritis.

*"Despite the scepticism of the traditional medical profession there is no longer any real doubt that this technique does work."*

For many years there was some confusion about how acupuncture works but today there are a number of acceptable theories.

It seems, for example, that at least two things happen when a needle is pushed into the skin. First, by introducing a sensation into the skin which passes along the larger nerve fibres and closes the gate in the spinal cord (see the explanation of the gate control theory on page 68), acupuncture is capable of preventing pain signals from reaching the brain. And second, when the acupuncture needles are pushed into the skin they also stimulate the production of endorphins (the human body's own pain relieving hormones).

Some scientists now claim that it is no longer necessary to follow the traditional acupuncture meridians in order to obtain a useful effect. It is, they argue, possible to obtain the same pain-killing effect by stimulating virtually any point on a fairly large area of skin.

In the past it was often claimed that if acupuncture didn't work it was because the acupuncturist had failed to 'hit' the correct acupuncture point. Today, it appears that it may just be that the patient was not one of those who was receptive to help by acupuncture.

The most dramatic development in the use of acupuncture was probably the fairly recent discovery that it is possible to obtain a type of acupuncture effect without sticking any needles into the skin at all. It is, it seems, perfectly possible to close the spinal cord gate and simulate the production of the vital endorphin hormones simply by applying heat or electrical stimulation to the body (by, for example, using a TENS machine – see page 68), or even by applying simple finger pressure to tender pressure points (this technique, which is not a new one, is usually known as shiatsu or acupressure and is becoming steadily more popular).

## ACUPRESSURE

Some historians believe that when acupuncture meridians were first mapped out practitioners did not use sharp needles but used their fingers instead. They argue that the needles so beloved of acupuncturists were only introduced to give the therapist the feeling that he was really doing something – and, perhaps, to make the charging of a fee more appropriate.

Acupuncture without needles but with fingers is usually called acupressure (though a variation of it is called shiatsu). As with acupuncture the aim is to restore the flow of energy along a meridian pathway when there is a blockage and to bring energy into the system when, for some reason, the meridian is empty.

In order to obtain a useful effect during acupressure the therapist presses quite hard on specific parts of the patient's body, using only his or her fingertips. It is, apparently, important to press quite hard. Some therapists claim that the therapist needs to exert a downward pressure of around 10 lbs (4.5 kg). If you try this out on a set of bathroom scales you will see that this is quite a lot of pressure.

Different therapists seem to use different pressure points and there does not seem to be a great deal of agreement between different acupressure specialists about the best points to use in order to treat specific conditions effectively.

The most effective acupressure points seem to be on or around the head and neck. By using finger massage at the top of the spine, on the centre of the cheeks, on the outer edges of the eyes and on the centre of the forehead between the eyes it is, say the experts, possible to relieve a wide range of symptoms. Another acupressure point is the one in the fleshy web that lies between the thumbs and forefingers of both hands. Massaging the acupressure point here is said to be particularly useful in the treatment of pain.

Because acupressure is a non-invasive, gentle therapy, it is said to be comparatively safe but I would recommend that if you want to try this form of treatment you consult a well-trained expert. Acupressure is said to be extremely useful in the treatment of arthritic pain.

## HYPNOTHERAPY

The Egyptians were fascinated by hypnotherapy several thousand years ago and then, for quite a long while, this speciality virtually disappeared from view. Then, in the 17th century, a man called Athanasius Kircher played around with the idea for a while. It was, however, a man called Franz Mesmer, who worked in the 18th century, who really brought hypnosis and hypnotherapy back into vogue.

The first evidence that hypnotherapy could help patients who were suffering from pain came from work done in the middle of the 18th century by a surgeon called James Esdale. Esdale made the extraordinary claim that he had performed 300 major surgical operations in India using hypnosis as the only anaesthetic.

During recent years hypnotherapy has come back into fashion again, and today there are many people who claim that it is a good way to deal with pain in general and arthritis in particular. Studies have been done which have shown that hypnotherapy can be used to increase both the pain threshold (the point at which pain is felt) and pain tolerance (the amount of pain that an individual can put up with).

Sadly, today there are many hypnotherapists around who have not (to be polite) received a very exhaustive training and there are some professionals who worry that the services offered by these practitioners may prove dangerous. If you think that you would like to try hypnotherapy as a way of combating the pain of your arthritis, I would recommend that you talk to your own doctor and ask him to arrange for you to see a professional and fully qualified hypnotherapist.

## HEALING

The difference between 'healing', 'spiritual healing' and 'faith healing' causes some confusion. Opposite, however, are the definitions which are commonly used:

1. **HEALING: THE WORD IS USED TO DESCRIBE THE WHOLE PHENOMENON OF HEALING WITH MEDICINES OR WITHOUT ANY OBVIOUS INTERVENTION BY THE HEALER**

2. **FAITH HEALING: THE PATIENT TRUSTS THE HEALER AND THERE IS A POWERFUL LINK BETWEEN THE PATIENT'S MIND AND HIS OR HER BODY**

3. **SPIRITUAL HEALING: THE PATIENT MAY OR MAY NOT KNOW THAT THE HEALING IS TAKING PLACE. HE MAY OR MAY NOT BE RECEPTIVE. THE HEALER TRANSMITS ENERGY FROM HIMSELF TO THE PATIENT IN SOME WAY.**

One of the most famous places at which healing commonly takes place is Lourdes, a town in the French Pyrenees which attracts around four million pilgrims a year — of whom about 65,000 are registered as officially 'sick'. Since 1858 a total of 6,000 people claiming to have received miraculous cures have been examined and 64 of them have been officially recognized as 'miracles'.

Despite the popularity of places like Lourdes, most healers claim that healing isn't necessarily mystical. They say that it does not have to be associated with religion of any kind.

Healers work in a variety of different ways. Some healers lay their hands on their patients. Others hold their hands above the patient's body. And there are healers who claim that they can heal someone without seeing him or her or, indeed, being anywhere near him or her. Some healers encourage patients and relatives to take part in the process of healing. Some talk or pray and some are silent.

A number of experiments have been conducted to show the effectiveness of healing. For example, in one Canadian experiment, it was shown that barley seeds which were made 'sick' by putting them into a saline solution would recover more speedily if they were touched by a healer. In America, Dolores Krieger, Professor of Nursing at New York University, has run controlled trials in

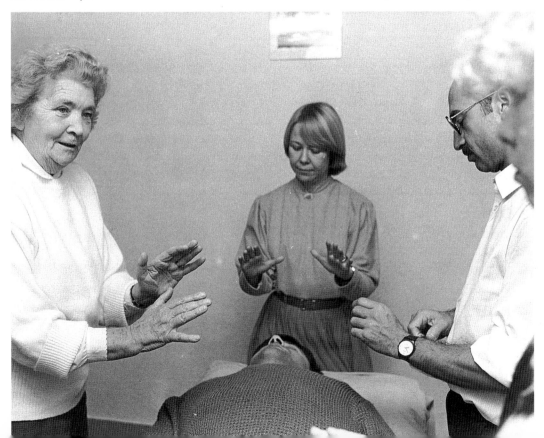

which she has demonstrated that blood changes produced by healing can, in fact, be measured and substantiated in the laboratory.

Healing can be used for just about any condition and there is no doubt that many patients with arthritis have benefited from receiving treatment from a healer. The majority of healers do not charge a fee for their services.

## ALEXANDER TECHNIQUE

The Alexander Technique is built around the idea that the condition and positions of the bones of the spine and the rest of the skeleton have an influence on our health.

The Alexander Technique, or Alexander Principle as it is also sometimes known, was first devised nearly a century ago by an Australian actor called F. Matthias Alexander. Mr Alexander noticed that he kept losing his voice when working on stage, and when the medical profession failed to help him he decided to try to investigate and treat his problem himself.

He realized that he was losing his voice whenever he was holding his head and neck in a particular position. He surmised that the voice loss was caused by the fact that the position of his neck was squashing his vocal cords.

After experimenting for several months he found that by learning to stand properly, and hold his head up straight, his voice no longer kept on disappearing.

So delighted was the actor by this discovery that he retired from the stage and decided to spend his life helping other people conquer their health problems by learning to stand correctly. He believed that just as his voice loss had been caused by poor posture so many other common illnesses might have a similar cause. Alexander's hope was that he would be able to treat problems which had already developed and prevent problems developing in the future, simply by teaching a few basic principles of posture and movement.

And so the Alexander Technique – an educational system designed to help teach people body self-awareness, graceful movements and good posture – was created. The aim is to find a patient's bad habits and get rid of them before any real harm is done.

Alexander claimed that people who stand upright and with their heads held high will have their internal organs in the right positions. He argued that such individuals would be far less likely to develop illnesses than individuals who slumped or sat and walked with a poor posture. He claimed that by improving posture and movement patients would be able to improve their digestion, their breathing and their circulation.

Modern followers of F. Matthias Alexander teach patients to move comfortably and to use their bodies properly. The technique is recommended to patients suffering from a wide range of problems but patients with disorders which involve the bones, the joints and the muscles seem particularly likely to benefit.

Individuals who want to benefit from Alexander's discoveries are encouraged to start by looking critically at the way that they sit, stand and walk, as well as the way that they lift and do ordinary, daily jobs around the house.

Followers of F. Matthias Alexander claim that every aspect of an individual's life should be examined. They say that even ill-fitting shoes can create problems. Sore feet can, they say, affect the way that an individual walks and so end up producing serious spine and joint problems.

## HOMOEOPATHY

No one really knows how homoeopathy works, but there are thousands of patients who believe that it does. The risks of side effects developing certainly seem to be slight and today, in an era when doctor-induced illness is commonplace, such an advantage is a fairly major one!

Although homoeopathy can be traced back for centuries, modern homoeopathy was first developed by a man called Samuel Hahnemann, who practised in the early part of the 19th century.

Hahnemann was rather unhappy about the medicines which were available for general medical use at the time. He knew that too many

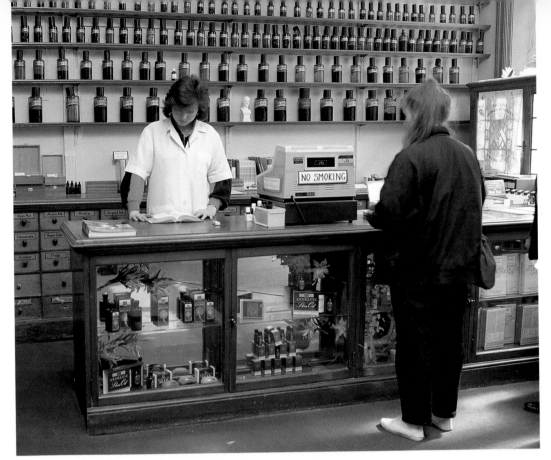

*A shop selling some of the 3,000 substances now available to homoeopaths.*

patients were made ill by being given large doses of potentially lethal products and he was, therefore, keen to find a method of treating people that would dramatically reduce the chances of a practitioner doing more harm than good.

Hahnemann knew that both Hippocrates, the father of medicine, and Paracelsus, the man who is widely credited with bringing medicine out of the dark ages and into a scientific era during the Renaissance, had believed that a patient can be cured if he can be given a medicine which will produce symptoms that are the same as the ones produced by his illness. This ancient theory was known as the theory of 'like curing like'.

Although he did not suffer from the ague Hahnemann decided to try to produce the symptoms of the disease in himself. By doing this he was following a long tradition of medical researchers in experimenting upon himself.

He knew that cinchona bark, which contains the drug quinine, would relieve the symptoms of the ague and so he took some of the drug. He soon developed the symptoms of the disease – including the fever. When he stopped taking the drug the symptoms disappeared.

Using as his basic principle the theory that 'a substance which produces symptoms in a healthy person will cure those symptoms in a sick person' Hahnemann decided to try to find more substances which would produce the symptoms of disease. During the next few years he experimented with an enormous variety of substances including certain animal products, vegetable substances, salts and metals.

By the time of his death, in 1843, Samuel Hahnemann had tested and 'proved' the efficacy of 99 different substances and he had created the basis of modern homoeopathy. Even more important, he had found that he didn't need to use large substances of the medicines he had 'proved' in order to obtain a useful result.

In fact, he found that very small doses made his treatments extremely effective.

By the year 1900, just over half a century after

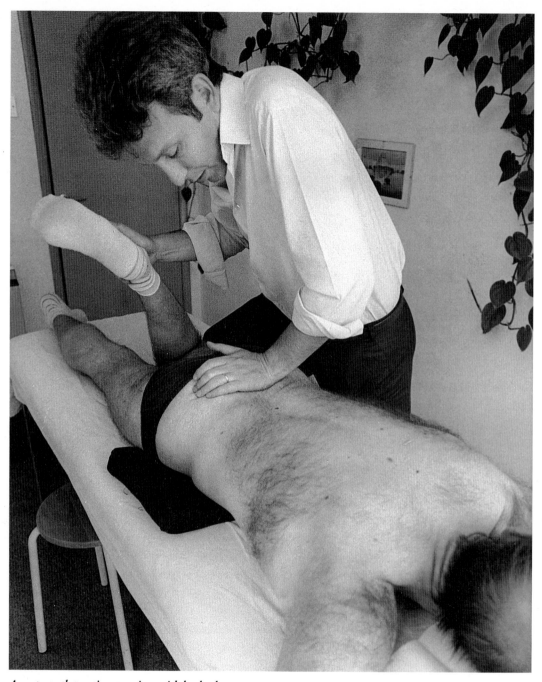

*An osteopath treating a patient with backache.*

his death, over 600 substances had been tested and found to have a useful effect. Today the number of substances available to homoeopaths is around 3,000 and includes honey-bee sting venom, snake venom, spiders, gold, copper, sulphur, mercury, onions and Indian hemp! Testings are still continuing in efforts to find more new substances which can be used in homoeopathy.

Making an accurate diagnosis is the first thing a homoeopath must do.

He or she will start by asking an enormous number of questions covering mental, physical and emotional issues which are designed to help the homoeopath find out as much as possible about the individual. The homoeopath will want to know about his patient's personal feelings, needs, anxieties and so on. He will also want to know how his patient responds to outside influences such as the weather and the temperature. In orthodox medicine doctors aim to treat diseases rather than patients, but in homoeopathy the treatment must be designed to fit the patient.

Having made a diagnosis the homoeopath will then choose a suitable 'medicine' from the list of 3,000. Homoeopaths usually try to find one medicine, however many symptoms a patient has.

The substance which is finally selected will be given in a very small dose diluted many thousands of times because homoeopaths believe that the smaller the dose the more powerful the response will be. Very small doses are used to trigger a reaction within the body. There are some similarities between homoeopathy and vaccination. In vaccination a small amount of an infective organism is given to the patient to get the body's natural defence mechanisms to start to operate. In homoeopathy a small amount of a drug is given in order to achieve a similar effect.

The doses which homoeopathic practitioners use are so incredibly small that they effectively put a drop of concentrated medicine into a bath full of water – and then use a few drops of the bath water as medicine!

Homoeopathy does seem to be very safe. But if you want to try this form of alternative medicine you should, of course, consult a properly qualified practitioner.

## CHIROPRACTIC

Chiropractic is based upon the beliefs formulated by a Canadian called Daniel David Palmer towards the end of the 19th century. Palmer held the extreme view that an extraordinary 95 per cent of illnesses were caused by displaced vertebrae (the technical term he used for displacement was 'subluxation').

These days, chiropractors take a less all-encompassing view of their technique. Many only deal with disorders of the bones and joints.

Using X-rays, they investigate parts of the body's frame that are displaced and pressing against nerves, causing pain. Treatment usually involves manipulation, done with the hands.

As with the other alternative therapies discussed in this chapter, it is important to consult only qualified and experienced practitioners.

## OSTEOPATHY

Although there undoubtedly are some osteopaths around today who claim that they are able to treat as full a range of diseases as a traditionally trained, allopathic doctor most osteopaths spend most of their time dealing with bone and joint problems.

Over half of the patients visiting osteopaths have backache and the majority of osteopaths seem to spend their working lives trying to help patients with back troubles, headaches, neck pains and joint pains of one sort or another.

Some professional osteopaths actually claim that they are descended (in professional terms) from the very first surgeons and the bonesetters of 200 years ago.

But modern osteopathy was first developed in 1874 by an American called Andrew Taylor Still who was the son of a Methodist preacher. Still, who hated drugs and alcohol, believed that the human body could be treated as a machine. He believed that it was faults in the musculoskeletal system which were responsible for many diseases.

Most osteopaths make an initial diagnosis by watching the way that their patients walk and stand and sit. They supplement these observations by talking and listening to their patients and by studying X-rays.

Osteopathic treatment usually involves a mixture of manipulation and massage.

It is vitally important to remember that osteopathy can produce problems and in order to minimize the risks you should only visit a practitioner who has been fully trained and you should make sure that he or she is well aware of your condition. There are many conditions – fractures, tumours, infection, inflammation and so on – which increase the chances of things going wrong.

# Aids For Arthritis Sufferers

*Because of stiffness in their joints, arthritis sufferers often have difficulty in walking, bending or reaching. The damage arthritis can do can be so severe that it can cause disablement and even crippling. To help overcome these problems there are many commercial products available. In addition there are many aids and gadgets which help to protect the joints and prevent the development of problems. The best aids will help you to make the most of all your remaining skills and will minimize the effect that your disabilities have on your life.*

*"The damage arthritis can do can be so severe it can cause disablement. To overcome this, there are many commercial products available."*

*Some arthritic patients are reluctant to use aids at all. They fear that to rely on any sort of assistance is to admit to a weakness; they even fear that it will speed up the disabling process. Nothing could be further from the truth.*

*The other fear, that gadgets and aids must inevitably cost a lot of money, is also ill-founded. There are, it is true, some pieces of equipment (particularly the electrical ones) which are expensive, but there are also gadgets which cost next to nothing and which can be made at home.*

*This appendix does not attempt to offer a comprehensive list of aids for arthritis sufferers but is designed to show the range of aids available. You should be able to obtain a full list of aids from your family doctor or hospital consultant but if you have any difficulty I suggest that you contact one of the many charitable or commercial organizations offering aids for the disabled. Big cities often have shops which specialize in equipment designed to make life easier for arthritis sufferers.*

## AIDS FOR SITTING

### POSTURE STOOL

The seat slopes forwards and you sit with your weight resting on your knees and your feet tucked in underneath you. The posture stool is especially designed to encourage you to sit in a healthier position with a better posture so that you can get up at the end of a day's work without having a stiff and aching back.

### BACKRESTS, 'WEDGES' AND LUMBAR SUPPORTS

The majority of chairs do not provide enough support for the lumbar part of the spine. You can obtain many different types of support – including inflatable cushions which are suitable for travellers – which will help turn your uncomfortable chair into one which is much friendlier to your back and other aching joints.

### ADJUSTABLE CHAIRS

Properly adjustable chairs that allow you to sit in a comfortable position are available, but they do tend to be expensive. The seat height should be adjustable, as should the angle of the seat and the backrest. You'll find it easier to get into and out of chairs which have arm rests that you can rest your weight on when sitting down or push against when standing up. If your feet aren't resting on the floor when you are sitting down you need to acquire a footrest because dangling feet add to the stress on your spine.

### EJECTOR CHAIRS

It is possible to buy chairs which, at the mere touch of a lever, help to push you up into the standing position.

## AIDS FOR WORK

### WRITING SLOPES

If you work on a computer, word processor or typewriter you may need to have a flat desk, but for handwriting you will find that a writing slope enables you to work at an angle which is better suited to your body.

## TIP FOR SURVIVING AT WORK

Get up and walk about every half hour. This will give you a chance to stretch your back and will help prevent muscle, joint and ligament strain.

## AIDS FOR PICKING THINGS UP

Simple 'pick up sticks' (such as are used by park attendants to pick up waste paper) help make life much easier if you find it difficult to bend or to reach for small objects. Pick up sticks are probably the most versatile and useful of all gadgets for the arthritic and disabled, yet they are basically nothing more than a pair of tongs with a long handle. They are also useful for drawing curtains, switching on lights, pulling on socks and doing a thousand and one other potentially painful chores. A pick up stick will extend your reach by 3 ft (90 cm) and enable you to pick up all sorts of things (clothes, newspapers etc.) off the floor without bending down. It is possible to buy sticks which fold up (so that you can carry them around with you) and some sticks have magnets on the end to help pick up metal objects.

## AIDS IN THE KITCHEN

If you have arthritis in your hands or wrists you will almost certainly find that one of the most useful aids available is a small device which will help you to open a jar. There are also aids to assist you to lift a heavy kettle or open a can (wall-mounted can openers are sometimes helpful). Some useful aids can easily be made by anyone with a few basic carpentry skills.

Preparing food can be tricky but the patient with only one useful hand will find that a spiked board will enable him or her to keep vegetables still while they are being peeled and chopped. To open packets it may help to stand them upright in a kitchen drawer, close the drawer as far as it will go and then cut the top of the packet open with a knife or scissors. Kitchen tools are easier to get hold of if they are hung neatly on hooks rather than placed inaccessibly in drawers. Cutlery should have large handles and you can adapt it to make it easier to use by wrapping tape around the handles or attaching bicycle handlebar rubbers.

One of the simplest and most useful gadgets you can buy if you have arthritic hands is a 'grip mat' – a small, non-stick rubber mat that can be invaluable for opening jars, bottles or even doors that are stuck tight.

If you are planning a new kitchen think carefully about the height at which you have cupboards and electrical sockets placed (it is possible to buy electric plugs fitted with handles – these are much easier to pull out and push in than ordinary household plugs). Try to make sure that everything you need is within easy reach and remember that taps are easier to turn on and off if they are of the lever type.

## AIDS IN THE BATHROOM

If you have arthritis in your hands you will probably find it difficult to operate ordinary taps so long-handled, lever type taps (the sort used by surgeons in operating theatres) can be a tremendous help. Alternatively you can obtain taps which can provide either hot or cold water with the same lever. A liquid soap dispenser which can be operated either by a foot pedal or a lever will make washing much easier. If holding a nail brush is difficult, one can be fixed to the side of the wash basin by screwing suction cups on to the back of the brush and sticking the suckers on to the basin.

As far as the bath is concerned one of the most important aids is probably the bathrail or handrail. A rubber mat in the bottom of the bath will prove useful for anyone who is slightly unsteady. People who find it difficult to lie down may be better off with a seat or board placed firmly across the bath. A lift suspended over the bath may be helpful (all sorts of hoists are available) and there are even special baths in which the bather sits rather than lies.

There are many other useful gadgets for the bathroom – sponges with long handles, tap-turners, long-handled brushes, toothbrushes with built-up handles and so on. Often it is not necessary to buy an aid – a home-made improvisation will prove equally effective. For example, it is possible to make a tap-turner with a piece of wood that has a hook fastened on to it and the handle of a toothbrush can be built up to a more manageable size either by wrapping pieces of sticking plaster over it or by fitting a bicycle handlebar rubber on to the handle.

As with everything else, it is best to isolate the problems first and then look for the solutions, which will often be quite simple. For example, someone who finds it difficult to operate a bathroom pull switch may find it easier if a ball is tied on to the end – one of those 'air' balls that golfers use for practice will be easy to tie on.

There are things that can also be done to make the other vital piece of bathroom equipment – the lavatory – more accessible. The toilet seat can be raised so that the stiff person does not have so much bending to do. It may be a good idea to have a small platform over the top of the toilet. And soft absorbent loose leaf tissue is easier to handle than a continuous roll. Finally, it is always wise to have several grab handles near to the lavatory, which should be very well secured.

## WALKING AIDS

Many arthritic patients are reluctant to use a walking stick because they think of it as a badge of infirmity. It should be regarded as an aid to walking – just as good shoes are an efficient walking aid. There are many different types of stick available, ranging from the ordinary wooden stick (which should have a rubber-tipped end to ensure that it does not slip) to the tripod type of stick. This has three feet attached to a single handle and will stand up by itself – it gives a bit more security than an ordinary stick and is almost as portable.

A walking frame is held in front – usually with both hands. When moving, the right and left side of the frame are shuffled forwards alternately. The frames are usually made of light but strong material and one major advantage is that a basket can be attached to the front so that small items (books, shopping etc.) can be carried around without having to use the hands. Some walking frames can also be converted into seats.

When choosing a stick or frame, do make sure that it is the right height. Frames usually have adjustable handles and sticks should be tried out for size. Some collapsible sticks and frames can also be obtained.

A stick or frame can give you extra support, take some of the strain and enable you to rest when you need to. If you use a stick, make sure you change hands regularly so that you don't get into the habit of putting too much strain on one side of your body.

## WHEELCHAIRS

There are many different types of wheelchair, so when selecting one you need to know exactly what you are going to use it for. Wheelchairs can be divided into three main groups: those most suitable for outdoor use, those suitable for use indoors and those which can be used either indoors or out of doors. Decide whether your chair will be pushed or propelled from inside. Look for a chair that is manoeuvrable and, ideally, collapsible so that you can take it with you when you travel by car, train or bus. Some chairs have detachable armrests and hinged footrests which make them a good deal easier to use because you can get in and out of them without exerting yourself too much .

Propelling wheels (the bigger wheels that the occupant moves to set a chair in motion) are usually at the rear but if you have limited shoulder movement you may get on better with a chair which has the propelling wheels at the front. Pneumatic tyres are more comfortable – particularly when you are moving over rough ground – but solid tyres make a chair easier to move and they do not puncture.

If you are going to use your wheelchair over long distances you may get on better with a powered model. There are many varieties of these available, some suitable only for indoor use, some suitable for use on quite rough ground. It really is a good idea to shop around – but first, make sure that you know what you want.

## AIDS FOR SHOPPING

If you have to carry heavy loads around use a shopping trolley or basket on wheels to relieve the strain on your back. Recent research from France showed that the average six-year-old French child regularly carries 9 per cent of his or her body weight in a rucksack or satchel while travelling to and from school. By the age of 12 the load has risen to 25 per cent and by the time they reach 16 years of age pupils are carrying 50 per cent of their body weight around with them in books, sports gear etc. It is hardly surprising that in the last decade the number of French citizens suffering from severe back problems has risen from 30 per cent to 45 per cent.

## AIDS FOR GETTING UP AND DOWN STAIRS

If you find walking up and down stairs painful you may find it easier if you edge yourself up or down on your bottom. If your problem persists investigate the possibility of installing a powered stair lift. You sit down on a small chair, press a button and ascend or descend the stairs without any further effort.

## AIDS FOR GETTING DRESSED

If you have difficulty in bending or raising your arms you will find that some clothes are far more difficult to get into and out of than others. Avoid tight jeans or trousers. Wear slip-on shoes rather than lace-ups. Make sure that zips and buttons are easily accessible and replace difficult to reach and tricky fasteners with easier ones. (Velcro fastenings are easy to close and undo.) Buttons, when you do use them, should be as large as possible. The long-handled shoe horn, the shoe which has an elasticated front and the long-handled pick up stick (see above) can all help. For women, a wrap-around skirt is easier to put on than one that has to be pulled up, while a front-fastening brassiere can be a great help.

Disposable underwear, towels and handkerchiefs may be expensive but do cut down on washing and ironing.

## TIPS FOR DRESSING

• Leaning against a wall will give you stability when you need to raise a foot or leg (e.g. to put on a sock or tie a shoelace).
• Roll up clothes such as jumpers so that you can put your arms through the armholes as easily as possible.
• If you have difficulty in balancing or pulling on trousers or tights try dressing while you are lying on top of your bed. To get your trousers over your feet, pull your knees up to your chest, then straighten your legs to pull your trousers up to your bottom.

## IN THE CAR

If you find you have difficulty in driving an ordinary car you should look at the possibility of having one 'customized'. You can buy better car seats and backrests to make sitting in a car more comfortable. Wide-angle mirrors make driving safer if you have only limited movement in your neck. There are also special knobs available which can be attached to the steering wheel to make steering easier.

## HOUSING: GENERAL ADVICE

Many of the minor hazards which the perfectly fit take in their stride can become major problems when joints stiffen and limbs don't work as well as they did.

For example, a flight of stairs which a fit and healthy individual can run up and down without any thought will provide an arthritic patient with considerable problems. Even a single high step or a couple of steps at the front door can suddenly become a restrictive barrier. High-rise blocks of flats where lifts may be out of order for months on end can turn into high-rise prisons for the disabled, and the lack of a ground-floor lavatory can mean a disabled person becoming marooned on the first floor.

Just as important as the type of home is where the accommodation is situated. A bungalow may seem a wonderful idea, but if it is at the top of a steep hill, hidden away in the country miles from a bus stop or railway station, or can only be reached by clambering up a steep path or a long flight of stone steps, it may be completely unsuitable for someone disabled by arthritis.

When you are planning a new home, or redesigning an existing one, it is important to be aware of the potential hazards and to think of future problems that might arise too. Uneven floors, steps between rooms and difficult passageways are all potential troublespots.

## AIDS FOR HOBBIES AND LEISURE

Just because you are arthritic you don't have to give up all your favourite sports and hobbies – there are many gadgets on the market that you can put to use.

If you enjoy fishing, for example, there are many special aids to help you hold your rod and cope with all your other equipment. If you like playing cards you can make a 'card holder' by sawing a suitably sized slit in a piece of wood. If you like reading but find it difficult to hold a book then put a tray with a small stand on your lap. If you enjoy sewing but have difficulty in threading a needle, buy a self-threading needle or an automatic threading machine.

For the arthritic gardener, there are plenty of useful tools available: long-handled gadgets for hoeing and weeding and picking up the rubbish, lawn mowers that can be operated from a wheelchair, spades and forks that can be used without bending and tools that can be used with just one hand for cutting long grass and pruning small bushes and trees. There are long-handled trowels, kneeler stools for gardeners with dodgy knees and all sorts of gadgets to make life easier in the greenhouse.

Finally, gardeners who have a lot of difficulty in bending can try building up their gardens to waist height. Walls of ordinary garden slabs are filled in with rubble and then good garden soil. Flower and vegetable beds can be separated by firm, even concrete paths. Raised gardens are even suitable for arthritics who have to do all their gardening from a wheelchair.

# ARTHRITIS INDEX

## PHOTOGRAPHIC ACKNOWLEDGEMENTS

The photographs in this book are from the following sources:
Arthritis and Rheumatism council, London 28;
Explorer, Paris/Jean-Paul Ferrero 67;
Format, London/Ulrike Preuss 118;
Sally and Richard Greenhil, London 111, 115;
Kobal Collection, London 81;
National Medical Slide Bank, Chelmsford 49, 64, 66;
Reed International Books: Peter Chadwick 117,
Rex Features Limited, London 72: Apesteguy/Sipa Press 40;
Tony Stone Photolibrary, London: Ken Biggs 34-5, Peter Correz 43, Andre
Perlstein 83, Rick Rusing 107, Philip Silcock 76;
ZEFA, London 13, 42: Kotoh 52, Madison 109.

### SPECIAL PHOTOGRAPHY
Richard Truscott  2, 4, 7, 17, 18, 23,24, 32, 45, 51,
63, 71, 77, 78, 84 – 87 (all), 93 – 105 (all)

### ILLUSTRATION
Kevin O'Keefe 91

Malcolm Chandler 36

Michelle Pickering 55

Jean Christian-Knaff 69

### LINE ARTWORK
Jared Gilbey 8 – 12(all)

ART DIRECTION Sarah Pollock

DESIGN Four Corners

EDITOR Sian Facer

PRODUCTION Simon Shelmerdine

PICTURE RESEARCH Judy Todd